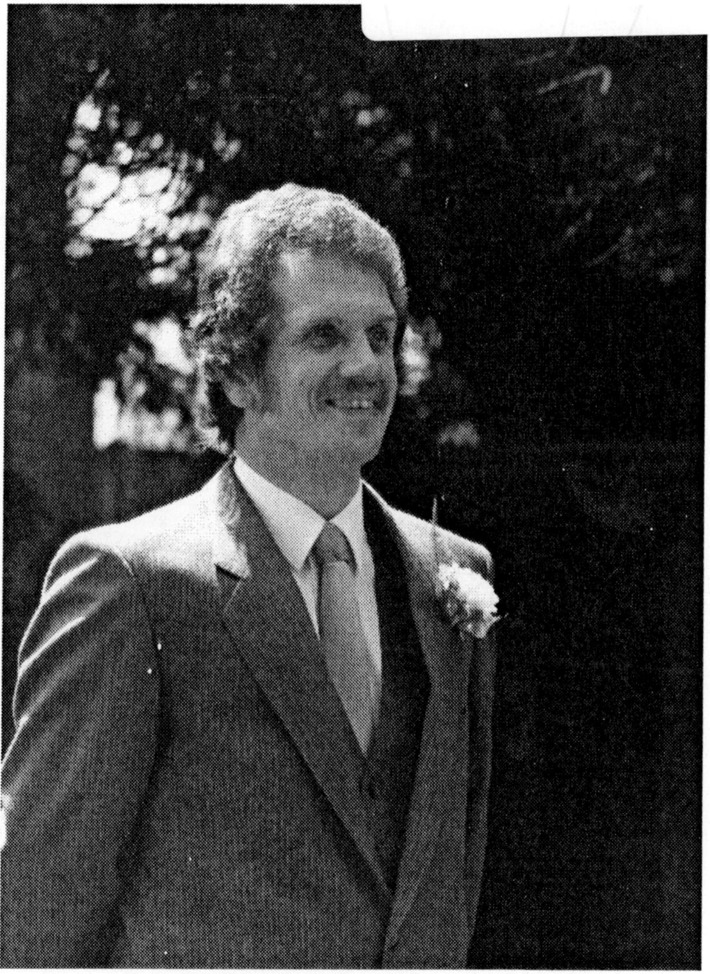

— *The author* —

ANOTHER WORLD

ANOTHER WORLD

Ian Litchfield

ATHENA PRESS
LONDON

ANOTHER WORLD
Copyright © Ian Litchfield 2004

All Rights Reserved

No part of this book may be reproduced in any form
by photocopying or by any electronic or mechanical means,
including information storage or retrieval systems,
without permission in writing from both the copyright
owner and the publisher of this book.

ISBN 1 84401 284 0

First Published 2004 by
ATHENA PRESS
Queen's House, 2 Holly Road
Twickenham, TW1 4EG
United Kingdom

Printed for Athena Press

A Split Second

On March 16th 1972 at 9.30 a.m.
I was sent to another world
No passport, no age limit;
I had to go… why, I do not know.

The reason for me to go I will never know
I do not think you could tell me why;
This world was like a child's world
I was to learn all over again.

I was as slow as a snail
I did so want to run but I just hobbled;
Walk correctly – never to be; I will always crawl like a snail
Speech – pathetic; you would think I was drunk.

Gosh, it was such a blow, a hefty blow –
To my parents it was such a blow!
A twenty-year-old son, the size of a man
The speed of a snail that could not keep up –
So embarrassing for all who were with me;
I felt so low and inferior, but I was going to win…

Acknowledgements

I THANK MY LATE FATHER, WHO STRUGGLED TO UNDERSTAND why I would never slow down. The reason – Father was such a hard worker; I was trying to follow in his footsteps. He died in January 1999. Thank you, Father, for never challenging my reason. Mother still lives on the farm. Thank you for the endless days of patience (most of the time), and thank you for those days when you drove me out into the countryside for me to escape the farm work. Mr Scott Ferguson was always there to advise me on my recovery plan. Thank you, Ruth, for the hard work in my bloody-mindedness, during my initial recovery in hospital.

Thank you to all the doctors and nurses who were involved in my recovery, and all my friends who helped me through my last thirty years, who have been kind enough to drive me from A to B and sometimes back to A. I would especially like to thank my friends in Madeira for giving the time to understand my speech and the weird shape I initially presented.

Preface

IAN LITCHFIELD WAS BORN ON 16 MAY 1953 AT BARRATT Maternity Hospital in Northampton. His birth was three weeks premature by Caesarean. Six weeks previous to his birth his mother had handled some chickens, which caused complications; hence this was the reason for the early birth.

Madeleine and Bob, his parents, owned a farm which was situated one mile outside West Haddon on the Yelvertoft Road. West Haddon is twelve miles from Northampton on the A428 and seven miles from Rugby. For those not familiar with the county of Northamptonshire, Ian's farm is situated three miles from Junction 18 of the M1.

Ian has a brother four years his elder. Both boys attended West Haddon Primary School from the age of four years till eleven years of age. The school which they attended from eleven years to fifteen years was Guilsborough Secondary School, which is situated three miles from West Haddon. From an early age Ian showed great interest in the livestock side of farming and his hobby at the age of fifteen years was rugby football. Phillip, his brother, preferred the arable side of farming at the age of seventeen years and his hobby was rally driving. Ian's school did not play rugby until his final year, which was 1968. Mr Haynes, the Physical Education Instructor, thought that Ian showed great potential and had mentioned him to the Rugby Club in the village in which Mr Haynes lived. His first game played was for Long Buckby Fourth Team. Long Buckby is a well-known rugger village due to the fact that it produced David Powell, who was an England International Player in the 1970s. The village over many years has produced some high quality teams. In his first game Ian played in virtually every position to see what he was capable of. He was a well-built young man, being five feet eight inches tall and twelve stone in weight.

Phillip had a much smaller frame, being only five feet seven inches, with a mass of light brown curly hair. He attended Moulton College of Agriculture at the age of seventeen years, one of the youngest students to attend college at this time as a live-in student. Ian attended day release classes at the Daventry Conservative Club; this was organised by Moulton College. Daventry was seven miles south of West Haddon. In the first year, Ian studied sheep and beef stockmanship, and machinery and arable farming. At the end of the year Ian passed his exams with flying colours. The second year he attended classes once a week at Moulton College.

His interest also included the Young Farmers Club. The club he chose to attend was Welford, as it was the nearest, being seven miles north of West Haddon. Part of the Young Farmers' activities included Stock Judging and Reared Calf Classes. Ian loved a challenge; the calves entered in the Reared Calf Classes had to be born at a certain time of the year and reared by the person exhibiting the calf.

What Ian enjoyed was planning when to start to lead and train the calf for the show ring. The calf is led with a halter, which is made of rope. The halter is placed behind the calf's ears and taken down to its jaw and round its nose. Sometimes for showing purposes the calf has a leather headpiece, similar to a horse's bridle. Training the calf requires application, strength and patience – all of which Ian had to offer.

At the age of seventeen years Ian had a reputation of being a promising rugby player. In the month of February 1972 Ian had been chosen to take part in the East of England Rugby Trials in the village of Long Buckby. In the trials, Ian had a wonderful afternoon and was selected to play for the East of England. Was this to be the start of an exciting life of rugby?

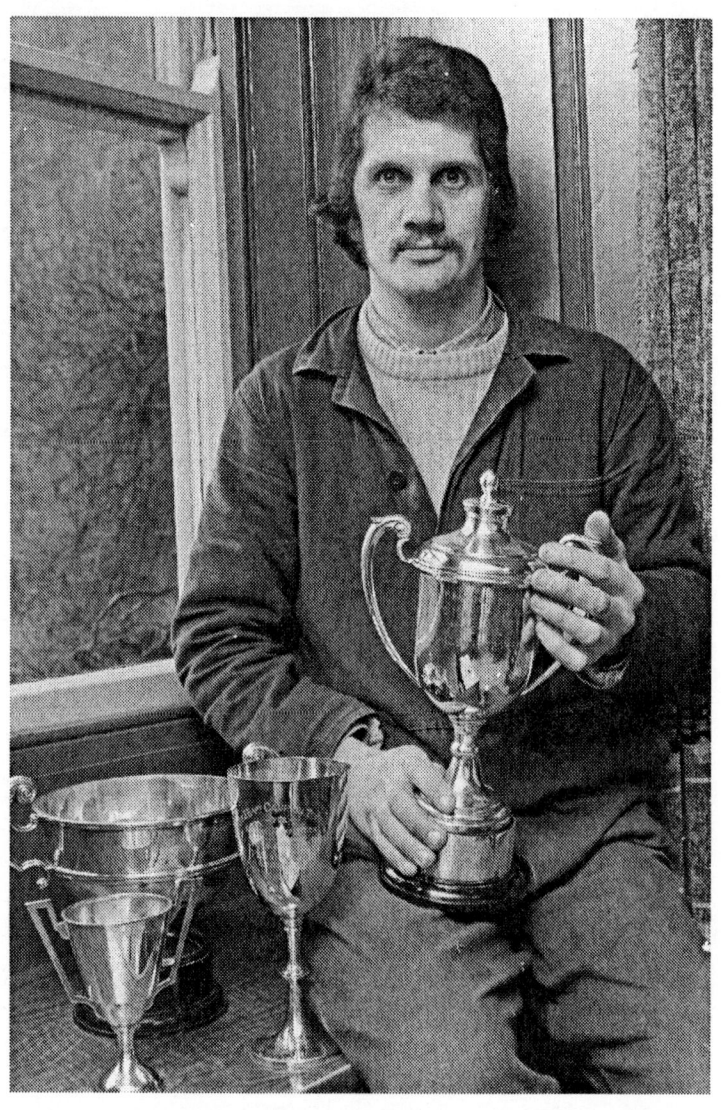

— *Ian with four trophies won in December 1982 with his lambs at Northampton and Rugby shows* —

Contents

A Split Second	vii
Acknowledgements	ix
Preface	xi
Chapter One ROUTINE	19
Chapter Two MOTHER'S FIRST NEWS	21
Chapter Three TUBES	24
Chapter Four THE FIRST CHANCE	26
Chapter Five MANFIELD	28
Chapter Six RIVERMEAD	30
Chapter Seven RETURN	33
Chapter Eight TALKING TO MY PARENTS	36
Chapter Nine ACCEPTANCE	38

Chapter Ten DERBY DYL	41
Chapter Eleven LIVESTOCK SHOWING	43
Chapter Twelve BOWLS	47
Chapter Thirteen JUST WORK	50
Chapter Fourteen SECURITY LIFE	54
Chapter Fifteen REFLECTIONS	58
Chapter Sixteen FEBRUARY	61
Chapter Seventeen EMOTIONS	64
Chapter Eighteen DRIVING	68
Chapter Nineteen RUTH	71
Chapter Twenty LAST CHAPTER	74
Chapter Twenty-one TOTAL SHOCK	76
Chapter Twenty-two MADEIRA	80

Chapter Twenty-three EMOTIONAL BREAK	86
Chapter Twenty-four MY NEW LIFE	90
Chapter Twenty-five HEADWAY	92
Postscript THIRTY-TWO YEARS	95

Chapter One
ROUTINE

THURSDAY, 16 MARCH 1972. THURSDAY WAS THE DAY OF the week I attended Moulton College, which was thirteen miles away depending on which route we took. It was my turn to drive. Jim, a farmer's son, and I used to share driving days. I asked Jim if he would drive. I had overspent on my father's petrol bill in his Wolseley 6/110, a very nice car with reclining seats. For the last six months I had been taking out a young lady called Jill from the next village, Crick.

My parents were not overjoyed with the friendship. This of course made me a lot keener. I had taken her out twice the previous week; my father was concerned about the amount of money I spent on petrol. I had plans for taking Jill out at the weekend. She was tall with long blonde hair – mind you, this came out of the bottle – and she had a lovely chuckle. Jill had just given me a cushion in the shape of a cat's head. This cushion was red. We named it Jake. Jill and I planned quite a night out that coming weekend. This would increase my father's petrol bill, which he would not appreciate. That was the reason I did not want to drive on this particular day to Moulton College.

The route to the college took us through West Haddon on the A428. Three miles out of West Haddon towards Northampton we turned left to East Haddon; we then took a road through the rambling countryside past a small village called Holdenby. Most of the village and land is owned by Holdenby Farms. We travelled another two miles to a village called Church Brampton. This village has a great quantity of houses due to its situation, as it is only a few miles from Moulton and Northampton. We then travelled over a gated level crossing and turned left; this took us up a slight hill for half a mile when we reached the top we came to the Market Harborough/Northampton main road. This was quite a well-known danger spot. After we had crossed the main road we went through Boughton village, which is a village of quality houses with horses and stables and small paddocks. The position and style of houses make it rather an exclusive area. Two miles further on we entered the outskirts of Moulton; we turned left onto the Pitsford road, and after a hundred yards we turned right into the college grounds.

In the Seventies the college's main education was in farming skills. Due to the turning tides of farming the college now offers lectures on many crafts; equestrian activities is one of the main crafts it teaches in the year 2002.

My father's routine each morning was to milk the twenty-one Friesian cows – these were the pride and joy of Father's farming. Phillip would have gone to our farm one mile away where he kept his pig herd; these were Landrace sows and a large white boar, which produce some wonderful meat pigs.

Mother's routine outside job was to fit the 250 hens kept in two large deep litters. A deep litter is a large wooden building which gives the hens plenty of area to roam in; the hens are also allowed to roam free outdoors, and this gave them a healthy life.

Chapter Two
MOTHER'S FIRST NEWS

16 March 1972 was a wonderful sunny morning. Routine was as usual at my farm home. In the kitchen, which is twenty-one feet long and nine feet wide, the walls were painted sea green. At the far end of the kitchen there was a dark green wooden gun rack which was on the brick wall, which was a light sea green. The floor was of old red and blue tiles.

Rachel, a friend of Mother's, a tall lady with blue eyes and dark short hair swept back behind her ears, had a wonderful smile and a quiet personality. She was visiting Mother, as she did each Thursday. My brother, Phillip, was also there with his mass of brown curly hair. Dick Payne, a neighbouring farmer's son, called my brother 'Curly'. Dick used to call me 'Beef' or 'Stout' – I think that speaks for itself.

My mother, who was fifty-three, five feet six inches tall, with a trim figure and a wonderful head of brown wavy hair, was washing up the breakfast crockery.

The phone rang. Phillip was two rooms away on the second floor. Rachel and Phillip were always fooling around – they each said the other could answer it. Eventually they both went. After about ten minutes they both returned.

Mother asked, 'Who was that?'

Rachel and Phillip looked at each other but made no attempt to answer.

'Come on, what is it?' Mother asked.

'About Ian,' replied Phillip.

'He has not cut himself, or something daft, has he? He hasn't been up town and knocked somebody off a bike or something?'

'No,' replied Phillip. By now Mother could see the white empty looks on Phillip's and Rachel's faces.

'No,' Rachel slowly and nervously replied, 'it is him that has been injured.'

Mother's First News

Mother went to the phone; they would not discuss anything but told her to get to the hospital straight away. Mother and Father went directly to hospital. Mother drove as usual; there was a lot of traffic in Northampton due to an accident on the M1.

When they got to Cheyne Walk, which would be 150 yards from the hospital, Mother jumped out and ran to the hospital building while Father parked the car. Mother entered the Accident and Emergency Ward. Keith Seargant, who was a fellow student, was there looking terrified. Mother said, 'Where is Jim?'

Jim was the person who was driving. He was at the Accident and Emergency door looking terrified. Mother asked, 'What's the matter?'

Jim said, 'He is very, very poorly.'

'He'll be okay,' Mother said.

Mother and Jim went into the Accident Department. Mother was taken to the George and Elizabeth Ward. There she was told I had a fractured skull, which did not worry her, as recently she had heard of somebody being discharged five days after receiving a fractured skull. She was not aware that this had only been a hairline fracture.

My condition was quite calm and I looked like a baby sleeping. Suddenly at 4 p.m. on Thursday afternoon I started to haemorrhage. This needed a large and very serious operation, which involved drilling five burr holes in my skull to relieve the pressure from my brain.

Six weeks after the accident Mother found out that on the day of the accident I would suddenly stretch my arms out and jerk and this would move my trolley down the corridor. While doing this I was having fits. This Mother heard from doctors explaining my serious condition to students from Oxford Hospital.

Father and Phillip were asked to be there at 6 p.m. on 16 March, so they were present for the operation as the chance of me surviving was very limited. Father and Mother stopped at hospital every night until 28 March. Keith, our farm labourer, milked the twenty-one cows morning and night. Friday teatime, the day after my accident, Mr Scott Ferguson told Mother and Father I would not live. Scott Ferguson, who was the surgeon operating on me, had a two-week holiday booked, but would stay if they wanted him to. A house doctor was in charge while Scott Ferguson was away. Scott Ferguson had said that I might live for three days due to my strong heart. If I lived till Monday I would need a tracheotomy to feed my fluids through.

Ten days after the accident Mother and Father left my bedside for the first time in the daytime. Mother bought some flowers for me as I, being a little romantic, always bought Mother some. 'It was the easiest thing to do.' I was the first patient to have flowers bought them in the ITU ward. Nobody had ever sat with a patient for such a long time as my parents did. Mother phoned in every morning to see how I was. She visited me at two o'clock every day, stayed till five, returned home to prepare the tea for the family and the workers, and returned at seven o'clock until twelve midnight.

One night, when Mother and the family were in the waiting room, Sister Walker came in and told Mother there were two young ladies, both with the name Ruth, who had been to see me. Would Mother try to find out who these young ladies were? One was Ruth Gowling, who was a nurse, a friend of mine; and the other was Ruth Tooley, a Young Farmers friend of mine.

Mother used to hold my hand and speak to me when I was unconscious. On the nineteenth day, in the afternoon, my eyes flickered. Mother called a nurse. For thirty minutes they watched, but flicker my eyes I didn't. Sister Walker thought that Mother had been wishing for my eyes to open. One hour later I squeezed Mother's hand. This was the first visible sign of life.

When Mr Scott Ferguson returned from holiday he could not believe I was still alive. 'What must his parents think of me?'

A nurse replied, 'They think you are wonderful!'

I kept looking at the clock but I could not see the hands, as I was virtually blind. Everything depended on my hearing. My mother organised a rota for visitors, morning, afternoon and evening. People rang home on the first weekend. All Father and Mother could say was the surgeon said that there was not a lot of hope.

Chapter Three
TUBES

I REMEMBER HEARING THE WORDS, 'IAN, CAN YOU HEAR? IAN, can you see? Ian can you hear? If you can hear, move your fingers!'

It seems as if I must have moved my fingers or finger, as I heard someone say, 'Quick, go and get the Staff Nurse.'

The next thing that I can remember is somebody moving my legs and arms. I then saw a mass of tubes and I pulled one out. It must have been from my throat, as I remember somebody saying, 'Put it back quickly.' It seems I had a reliance on the tube to feed me. I must have drifted in and out of consciousness as the next thing I can remember was being sat on a chair at the side of my bed. My mother was standing by my side. The next ten days seemed to be a little confused.

Next I remember passing through corridors for approximately ten minutes. I was on quite a shaky bed trolley, with a tall, dark, male nurse leading the trolley and a blonde, short, chubby little nurse pushing from the rear. We passed through two swinging blue doors; it was then I knew for the first time from viewing a sign on the wall that I was in Northampton General Hospital. Northampton Hospital is built with light brown bricks and is situated in the centre of Northampton between the Bedford and Kettering roads. The ITU ward, which I had been discharged from, was in the main block of the hospital. As we passed through the blue doors, it was instant sunlight; the road that we crossed was approximately six yards wide. This was a service road to car parks for the hospital. The building we were entering led to the George and Elizabeth wards. I reached those by entering a small lift that took me up to the wards. The George and Elizabeth wards were in a tall building with large paned glass windows. The remaining building was lower and housed the x-ray areas, the emergency facilities, out-patient rooms and cafeteria.

As I was pushed into the George and Elizabeth corridor, which was quite a dull blue colour, I was greeted by a cheeky smiling young lady named Ruth who was approximately five feet eight inches with short, dark curly hair and lovely blue eyes.

'Hello, Ian, come back to see us again?'

The young nurse had been on duty on 16 March when I was admitted into the Accident and Emergency section of the hospital. Ruth had been assigned to me to gain experience and also, as she was quite tall, she would enable me to walk with assistance. I later found out that she had a nice firm figure when my hand accidentally fell down off her shoulder. Oooohhh, aaahhh, that was quite comforting, I was alive again! The times she virtually dragged me along the corridors to encourage me to walk... What I really enjoyed was her assistance hauling me along the twenty yard corridor to the female section of the ward. I eventually found out that she had a completely nice figure and a lovely personality, which was helpful, as I needed encouragement. At this time I did not realise that the collision on 16 March would affect my entire future life.

Chapter Four
THE FIRST CHANCE

THE REASON RUTH HAD BEEN ISSUED AS MY NURSE WAS THAT she was the only nurse who was tall enough to be able to aid me to walk again. Clive and his sister – who were physios – also helped me very much. They both helped me in the ITU ward and the George and Elizabeth wards.

It was six weeks after the accident and I was not too sure why I was in hospital. The injuries I received when hitting my head on the door frame were very severe. It obviously did not do a lot of good to me. I was left with blurred vision, slurred speech and a paralysed left side. I did not feel ill; it was just like starting from being a child, with limitations, but with an eighteen-year-old's desires.

On Tuesday morning, when I was due for my regular bed bath, Ruth had a wonderful idea. It was time I had my first real bath. Ruth and an assistant walked, or should I say dragged, me to the bathroom. The bathroom was a plain blue room with not as much room as you'd need to swing a cat (well, I hadn't got a cat to swing!). Yes, the bathroom was quite small, the bath was one of the old type deep baths which, if you are not careful, you could drown in. Ruth submerged me in the warm bath. It was wonderful. I can remember it as if it was yesterday – or maybe it is memorable for another point. Ruth and her assistant were called back to the ward, for an emergency. While they were out I decided to stand up the first time ever since the accident happened, and dry myself. Well, as I struggled to stand up, I faced a mirror in the bathroom. What I saw was frightening – no hair! I did not realise it had all been shaved off. It was all a blur as my eyes were still like clots of blood. My body looked like an older person's body with no flesh. I just sank back into the bath with horror.

When I was eventually taken back to my bed, I lay down and looked back over my situation, not having realised what a mess I was. I had difficulty in making my left arm and hand work, and found it hard to swallow the food, now that they had taken the food tube out of my throat. I just did not understand. It was at this time, as my memory of the past was not affected, I decided my goal was to play rugby again. That goal I was to reflect on many times during the next thirty years. You must set a goal to achieve, to reach new levels of fitness. This gives you more respect for your body, and during periods of depression, makes you less ashamed of yourself. Also your ambition to reach fitness gains respect.

It was after viewing myself for the first time that I started to act differently to relatives and friends who knew me as the fit, active person never known to turn down a dare. I started to sink into being a solemn, not very talkative person. I thought wrongly; I should not be ashamed at being a poor reflection of my previous self. With people who I had not known previously, I was fine – even making jokes about being like Twiggy but with better looks. The big disadvantage with having a near useless left arm and hand. If you're using a urine bottle in the bed, you cannot get the bottle down in time and – oops – you end up with wet sheets and bed. That's when the aftershave comes in useful. The sheets dried out but the aftershave helped the fragrance.

There are stories about how you get rid of food you cannot manage to get on your spoon. I think I will leave that to your imagination. I am sure we have all done that in our younger days. (I was back to my childhood again.) Eating peas was a great challenge as you can imagine, following the peas around your plate. My peas always seemed to be cunning, and they either ended up on the floor, in my bed or down my pyjamas. My left arm and useless hand proved to be an obstacle forever to overcome. At this point, I decided that any challenge was worth taking on. In fact my life had become a total challenge in this new world of mine. Every day of my life I will have my slow leg, painful when any strain's put on it, and my slow bent arm. Will my hand ever work again? Will my movements always look like those of a child? Will my body ever mature into that of a respectable-looking human?

My lifelong challenge and goal was to regain my physical stature, gain people's respect and not feel inferior.

Chapter Five
MANFIELD

AFTER SEVEN WEEKS AT THE GEORGE AND ELIZABETH IT WAS decided by my surgeon, Mr Scott Ferguson, to move me to a hospital on the outskirts of Northampton for a rehabilitation period. Mr Scott Ferguson was on duty on the 16 March 1972 when I was admitted to Northampton Accident Ward. I had to undergo an operation after haemorrhaging of my head. Throughout the past thirty years, Scott Ferguson has been wonderful. As soon as I have contacted him for advice or to complain, he has made himself readily available. He is now semi-retired.

Manfield House was built in the late 1800s in a Jacobean style, with Northamptonshire stone. In fact, the building was built for a Mr Manfield, the owner of Manfield shoe manufacturers. Mr Manfield gave Manfield House to the health organisation for the treatment of limb diseases in children. The house, renamed Manfield Hospital, was also used for tuberculosis.

The wooden wards were added in the grounds of Manfield House for the treatment of people with tuberculosis, as this was one way of controlling the disease – in a park-like setting with frequent visitors – the grey squirrels – often in attendance.

At the same time as I was moved to Manfield, my nurse, Ruth, had been sent to Manfield Hospital to get experience as she was only a trainee nurse. 'My nurse' – that sounds selfish – was then moved to the same hospital in the position of assistant, but unfortunately not on my ward.

As soon as I became conscious after the accident and started to put weight on my left leg, I suffered severe pain in my thigh. Countless x-rays revealed nothing. The only damage my clothing received in the accident was a slight tear on my jeans on the left knee. The new hospital was quite a contrast to my past ward. Whereas in my last ward I had constant help, in this ward I had to fend for myself.

With the aid of a walking frame I started to walk, or should I say stumble. Within two weeks I was chief tea-trolley controller. Good fun! I could meet all the new patients and the young trainee nurses. Life was becoming interesting. I received physiotherapy everyday to my legs and arms, which was very tiring. My left arm was still partly bent and my left leg was very weak. I was ashamed of my body and my coordination. At the end of May it was apparent that I needed a lot more physiotherapy, more than they were able to give me at Manfield. It was decided to move me to another rehabilitation hospital on the outskirts of Oxford. I have found out since that I had been quite a handful for the nurses and doctors with my mood swings, and I became so independent and uncontrollable that I had organised my own transfer to Oxford Hospital, leaving the nurses to tell my parents I had gone.

Chapter Six

RIVERMEAD

It was a long sunny drive to Rivermead Rehabilitation Hospital on Abingdon Road on the outskirts of Oxford. It's seventy miles approximately from Northampton, depending on which route you take.

The Rivermead Rehabilitation Hospital was set in a lovely semi-rural area. As you entered the driveway there was a new ward on the left, which was for the new female and male patients. Further on there were two brick buildings, one for the improving female patients and the other for the confident and improving male patients. These wards were used to rehabilitate the patients' self-care abilities. Further to the left of the building were the gym and swimming pool, and to the right of these was a handicraft building. At the far end of the hospital grounds was a tributary to the river.

The first person who I met at Rivermead Hospital was Gerry. He was five feet nine inches with fine light brown hair. He had a pale complexion with an infectious smile. He was confined to a wheelchair. He had a wonderful wife named Bernie and a son, Vincent. Although Gerry had a lack of speech he had a fantastic personality – I can honestly say we had four months of great laughter.

There was a pub called the Black Horse 300 yards away. I was allowed to push Gerry up to the pub in the evenings. This was authorised as long as we did not drink alcoholic booze. The journey to the pub did us good as it gave us exercise and a chance to meet with other people.

The craft buildings I mentioned earlier were involved in woodwork and wicker making skills. These activities encouraged the patients to use their weak limbs, which gave them more confidence and strength. I have always liked woodwork when I had time. In the twelve months I was at Rivermead Rehabilitation

Hospital I made a wooden train. This was a great enjoyment to me, as I used an electric saw bench aided by my useless hand. I made a total of eight wooden trays with woven straw surroundings. As patients taking part in these skills, we were encouraged to use both our hands, which created more coordination.

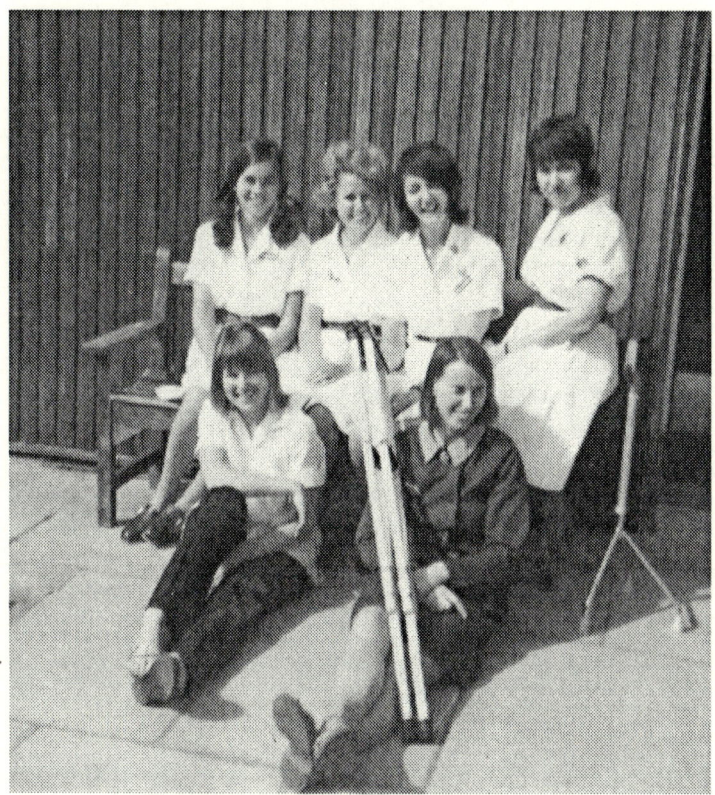

— *Physiotherapists at Rivermead Redabilitation Hospital* —

While I was there, I had a regular girlfriend visiting me on occasional weekends. It was only occasional weekends, as she needed to find somebody to drive her from her home eighty miles away. This was where life got complicated. At my regular visits to a shop nearby, I met a lovely young lady with a fantastic personality; her name was Jenny. She worked in the general-purpose shop opposite the pub that Gerry and I visited. Jenny had lovely shiny black shoulder-length hair, which she kept very smart, as she was an ex-hairdresser. Jenny and I became good friends. Life soon got difficult, as Jenny would visit me unannounced, which was quite a nice surprise, but it got a little complicated if she was visiting me when my regular girlfriend arrived. I began to think that life was worth living. I had to start to organise my life with ladies again. This was a challenge, and it was good for me to start to organise my situation, especially due to my brain-injury. My weight improved greatly, in fact I became slightly chubby, which was not a great help to my weak limbs and my coordination; but this started to improve over the following weeks. Control of my weight has been an ongoing task. I am seven pounds heavier now than at seventeen, not bad really.

Due to my uncontrollable moods and outbursts the hospital decided that a home visit might calm me down, as they could not control me. At this stage of my recovery I was going through an unmanageable period. The doctors and nurses could not control my fits of temper; their only conclusion was to send me home for one night, and hopefully this might control my temper, with the familiarity of my own home surroundings. My mind wandered back home. Not having been there for three months being able to see my parents in my own home… this surely would be wonderful.

'Yes,' I said, 'I would love to. I will see if my parents can arrange transport.'

During the following week, my mind went back to my large country home and enjoyment to see my family.

Chapter Seven
RETURN

MY PARENTS BROUGHT ME BACK TO THE RIVERMEAD Rehabilitation Hospital on the Sunday afternoon. My parents had collected me on the Saturday morning on the previous day. I was full of excitement, as were my parents. When we approached my home, the drive to my home was tarmac. The fields on either sides full of sheep. As we reached the bottom of the drive, which was 200 yards long, we entered a concreted farmyard. Thirty yards straight ahead of us was a silver iron gate that opened into a large grass field with a lake, two-thirds down in the field. The far left of the farmyard was a cowshed where you could milk twenty-one cows. To the right was a covered yard where you can house twenty-two cattle; to the left of the yard as you enter there was a small house yard enclosure that led to the kitchen. My home was next to the farmyard in which there were milking cows waiting to enter the milking parlour. Nothing on the farm was tidy the way I could remember. Buckets were not in the correct place. The concrete floor was not swept. The cowshed broom was lying on the floor rather than in an upright position. These things continually got me frustrated, as I could not cope with these minor jobs. To me they were awfully important. The accident had made me quite a perfectionist, or maybe I had time to see when things were out of place; but even these small tasks I could not cope with at the start of my farm work.

Getting out of the car was difficult, and stepping onto the step up into the small yard that adjoined the house, which took us into the kitchen, seemed to take ages to complete. The kitchen was large, and very tidy as my mother always used to keep it. Hell had just broken loose in my head. Everybody was trying to help me either up the steps or to sit down or to stand up. They wanted to pass me a plate, get me something to eat, make sure I ate, and many other frustrating incidents. I hid the frustration until the following day.

On the weekend I came home from Rivermead Hospital, the West Haddon Fête was held at the vicarage. I was determined to attend; Mother and Father were very concerned. I was going to show people that I was fit enough to take part in celebrations, mentally and physically. The trouble began when I approached a three-inch lawn edge – to me it was like climbing a two foot wall – but I completed that feat and continued to walk. Well, I moved as fast as an old snail, only not quite as straight! I believe it took me about forty-five minutes to go round the fête. When I returned home I felt so inferior, after seeing people of my own age running about, and from the fact I was totally exhausted. For the next five weeks my ability to achieve tasks disappeared and I sank into one of my first deep depressions. I could see no way out. My bouts of depression were quite serious for five years. You go so far back in your physical condition and mental state that it takes twice as long as your depression to regain your original state. At the time of your depression this fact does not enter your mind.

I had spent a sleepless night, frustrated by the way everybody wanted to help me, not giving me time to complete my tasks, as it took me a long while to complete them due to my lack of coordination. The jobs on the farm were not done as tidily as I would have completed them, and everything seemed out of place. Also my experience at the fête did not help. On Sunday morning, I exploded, I could not hide my frustration any longer. I said a great deal which ended in, 'Take me back to hospital!' Gosh, what my parents must have thought!

As we entered the hospital grounds, it was with great delight and relief. All was in the same order as I had left it. Gerry was there awaiting my return, he had his usual beaming smile. It would not be long before Jenny would be down to see me. Heaven at last. My parents fetched me home at weekends, except when my Uncle Cliff or other friends visited me; then they would transport me out of the hospital grounds.

After my weekend away, I was moved to the ward for improving patients. Life proceeded, and I became fitter, though my leg was still very painful and my speech often slurred. Within the next eight months I went home many times. Each time I returned to hospital depressed. Finally the decision was made to send me home, as they considered I was able to cope there. The doctors did not realise the turmoil my head was in. Could I cope with untidy property, jobs I was incapable of completing, and people in too much of a rush to help me? But I had to leave hospital, as they needed my bed for more patients requiring rehabilitation. Fond farewells were said, I had a farewell gift from my physiotherapist, whom I secretly had fallen in love with. We were all given our own personal physiotherapist, not one to one but five patients to one physiotherapist. This seemed to work very well. It was nice to tell people I had my own physiotherapist.

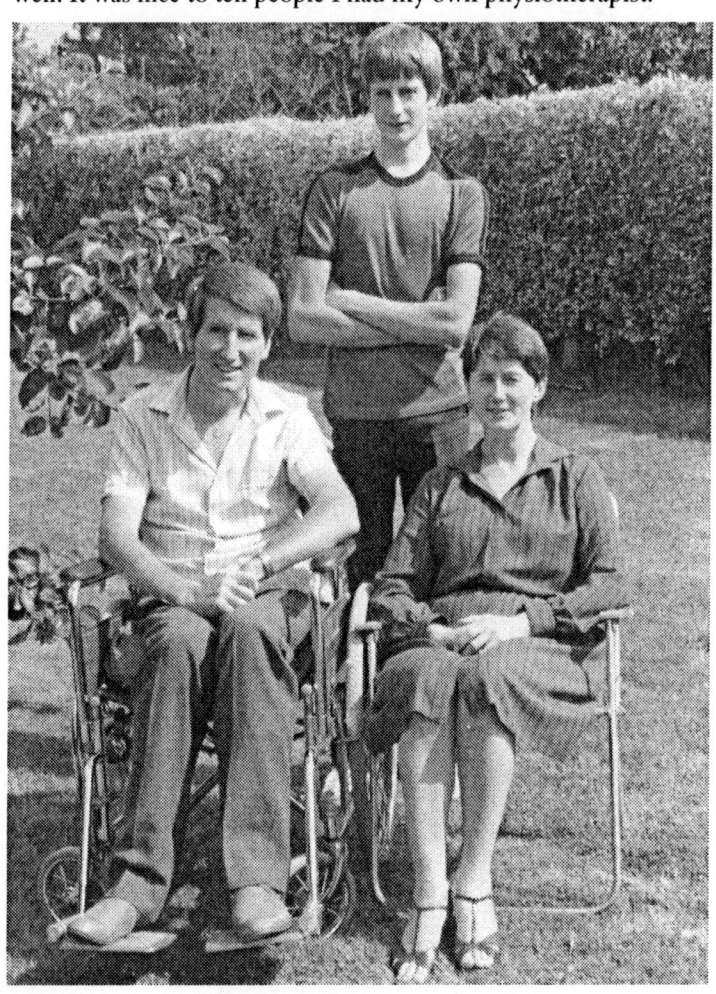

— *Gerry, Bernie and their son, Vincent* —

Chapter Eight
TALKING TO MY PARENTS

I HAD BEEN DREADING RETURNING HOME. WHEN MY FATHER came in from work, which was never before one o'clock at night, all year round, I decided to ask my father and mother to sit down and listen to me. What I said next must have given them great concern, not wanting me, in their view, to make mistakes and errors of judgement when carrying items or moving with little finesse.

I did not realise at the time. It must have been hard for them to agree to. Until my father's dying day he worried about me, but never stood in my way; my mother is still alive and has found it hard to keep quiet. What I told them was that I never wanted any physical help in doing anything, not even if I fell over. They should leave me and I would struggle up again. It made me feel so inferior to be helped and I must be given respect. I knew what was best for me, to struggle to reach perfection; if not this time I would try again.

Three months went by. I had to struggle with farm work. I could cope with 9 a.m. till 11 a.m. Then I'd have a snack lunch out, and persuade Mother we should visit someone who might have been a friend of Mother's or a friend of mine. This was just a way of getting away from the work I could not cope with.

The person who worked for my father, named Keith, unfortunately passed away at a young age with cancer. Keith had a country complexion, was not married and had an easy-going attitude to life. He was always a relaxing companion for me and he took nothing seriously. He was completely different from Father. With Keith's easy-going attitude, it helped me cope with my inability to complete my jobs.

After a few months, I could not handle my unfinished work, which was due to my weakness and the pain I was suffering in my left thigh. I applied for a position as progress chaser at Express Lifts, an engineering company at Northampton, which is twelve miles away from my home. This was a complete change of direction for me, but what appealed to me was the shortness of the working week, as on a farm you are required to work seven days most of the weeks. To my great surprise I was given the job. It took a little time to get used to the new situation but it was quite interesting as it involved meeting various people. After six weeks, I had to take leave from work because of the flu. I decided not to return to the job. Sitting down all the time might exercise the brain but not the body, which I needed to exercise constantly.

During the next six months, I had to make a decision, as my steady girlfriend asked if I would consider settling down with her. The answer was no. This meant I would be losing her lovely long legs that went to I don't know where, that lovely chuckle and that consuming smile, as I found it difficult to earn enough money for me to survive, let alone to have a second person to look after. After I'd made my decision, Jill went to live with somebody else. Life started to get lonely. I decided to work on my fitness rather than keep my social contacts. That was the worst decision I have ever made.

In 1974, after a winter of discontent due to being unable to fulfil my expectation of work given me, I decided to try working as a butcher's assistant at Baxters Butchers in the nearby town of Rugby, which was seven miles away. I tried very hard; I enjoyed the public contact and the variable work. But the continuous standing in the butcher shop played hell with my leg, so I was forced to finish this job.

Six months later, I became an assistant in a farm shop in Daventry. I think I still hold the record sale. This was for selling one tonne of hen's grit (when eaten, grit helps to form hard shells on eggs). I was getting on well with the shop, organising the top floor of the premises, and I was enjoying great contact with local farmers coming in to order or collect food. Unfortunately the manager disappeared from the shop and his home. At the start of my job, I had the understanding of the manager that I was not to be involved in any heavy lifting concerned with moving the food. The new manager expected me to carry bags of food all over the shop, up and down stairs. This did not suit my back, so again I had to resign.

Chapter Nine
ACCEPTANCE

Leaving the job at Daventry in the farm shop was a great disappointment. A friend from my rugby-playing days, Geoff Ridgeway, told me he was always a big believer in doing whatever you're good at. I don't think Geoff realised how despondent I got when I was unable to complete a job at work on the farm. I decided to accept the injuries, and the effect this had on me was an improvement on my completion of tasks. I was very stubborn (possibly due to the fact that I am born under Taurus). Once I accepted my situation and challenge, I had to win. I started to accept people's help, and I began to make progress on my fitness rehabilitation. The trouble with my situation was that my looks never got me any pity. Although I had a slow left side and my speech had greatly improved, I did not appear to be in as bad shape as I was. I once said, 'I wish my inside feelings showed outwardly.'

I kept everything to myself, as I don't think anyone really understands unless they have been in the same situation as I was. Every head-injury is different, and there was not an authority on head-injuries in those days. Physiotherapy is something I believe I should have continued after leaving hospital. Farm work is very strenuous and varied but doesn't always exercise the part of the body one needs to, to enable strengthening of the limbs. Hindsight is a wonderful thing; people were just so pleased I was alive. At several stages of my recovery I wished I was dead due to my lack of capabilities. I felt I was such an embarrassment to my family and friends.

I decided to go swimming at the local pool in the town of Rugby, which as I said is only seven miles away. I was allowed to drive three years after my accident, this meant I could be independent and take myself swimming. I believed, and was told by the physiotherapist, that the pool exercise would help my leg and arm, which indeed it did.

Something I forgot to mention: when I was released from Rivermead Hospital, I was only taking four tablets but now three years later due to bouts of depression I was on sixteen tablets a day – some to calm me down and some to boost me up. Well, I felt like a bloody yo-yo.

My daily routine was shepherding sheep and cattle. Shepherding entails driving or walking through fields where the sheep and cattle are kept, making sure that the total of stock are still in the same field and that the stock are not suffering any kind of illness such as watery eyes, and checking no animal has a severe attack of worms. The first indication of this would be an empty stomach showing a hollow gut or a dirty back end.

I accept the tablets eventually got into my system. One day as I came out from the field I had been shepherding onto the main road, there was a verge of five yards where I could park the Land Rover and could shut the gate I had just driven through. For, I believe, five seconds, I saw two gates; well, I thought the sun had affected me. I jumped into the driver's seat and turned right onto the main road, for half a mile I was fine and then to my horror, I saw two or three cars coming towards me directly in my path. I couldn't take to the grass verge to avoid these cars, as the verge had turned into a boundary wall running along the side of the road. I just braked and stopped; I did not have time to put the warning signs on. Thank God there was no close traffic following me. I just sat there for what seemed like minutes: probably it was just one minute. I drove half a mile back to a grass field and went across the field to home. Obviously the tablets were not the innocent party in the double vision I had just experienced. That was the last time I took tablets. Depression had to come and go.

Driving was my release from frustration and also it got me away from farm chores I could not cope with. If I had continued taking these tablets, I surely would have lost my driver's licence or run somebody over. Losing my driver's licence or not being allowed to drive on the road would have been taking my whole life away.

The Show Must Go On

I was dealt one large blow –
One most would not survive –
I did; why did I survive?
The show must go on

A goal you must decide,
Beyond you, never mind. Just try
Every step with that wonky leg.
A step towards recovery
The show must go on

To play bowls made my leg
And my head ache. My eyes became
Misty with confusion. My arm had to wake
The show must go on

My parents and friends looked on in disbelief
Every challenge was to show that my
Looks and disability did not stop one
Hundred per cent achievement.
Remember please that things are
Not always what they look, and
People's achievements are limitless –
God, the ruddy show must, must continue
On and on…
Thank you all for your patience.

8.45 a.m.
8 June 2002

Chapter Ten
DERBY DYL

IN 1978 I DECIDED THAT I NEEDED TO BE INVOLVED IN preparing and showing cattle again. Father and I decided to go to a cattle sale at Derby to purchase a beast that was good enough for showing. Show beasts for a prime stock show for butchers' requirements need to be a medium-length body with a good wide rump. They need to have a good short neck so as to avoid producing low value meat. The body should be covered with flesh, not fat. A bullock's (castrated male) flesh content has decreased in fat cover tremendously in the last twenty years. This is due to so-called 'expert' views that fat is not good for you. If your beast lacks fat you might as well be eating a wooden door, as it would have as much flavour. Actually I am not a great beef eater, mainly because I live on my own and I do not enjoy cooking.

We decided to purchase a cow and eight-week-old calf. The mother was a Charolais cross, Friesian mother; she was a red colour. This was in the single suckle section. 'Single suckle' means the cow only suckles one calf and therefore lays in the field with its calf – this creates a low maintenance expense.

Training the calf for showing can start at an early age of twelve weeks. Starting at this age requires a lot less power by the person who is training the calf. I was the one training the calf, and I had very little power at this short time from my accident.

The first thing we do is to put a halter on the calf's head in the same way as you place a headpiece on a horse. You then tie the calf to a solid tying point, this makes a calf respect the control of a rope halter. After about six episodes you then slowly walk the calf around an enclosed yard. You use an enclosed yard, as this stops the calf escaping if it gets away from you. After about two weeks I was able, well, the *calf* was able, to lead me up the roadway! At this stage I was hardly able to walk, after all the strenuous leading of the calf. This continued every other day for the next nine months. We were then able to take him to his first show. He really behaved very well and we gained second prize.

Time moved on, and after exhibiting him at many summer shows, we exhibited him at Blakesley Country show, a small show but with quality stock. These shows I preferred, as I could take the animal home with me, rather than take him to a prime stock show at Christmas and have him slaughtered. As he became older I found he was eating a lot of food and becoming quite expensive to keep. I then decided to take him to Rugby prime stock show at Christmas.

The effect of showing Derby Dyl at Christmas was heartbreaking. All his life he had gained trust in me and I had slowly taught him to respect the halter and trust me. Well, as I led him round the sale auction and finally released him after his sale, I inwardly was sick. How could I let poor old Derby Dyl be slaughtered after all the trust he had put in me? If I ever had a heart it was completely broken now. When I got home I cried my eyes out. The one thing the accident had done to me was make me feel very sensitive about animals putting their trust in me. I swore that I would never ever allow myself to be in the position with an animal that I have him slaughtered after putting so much faith in me.

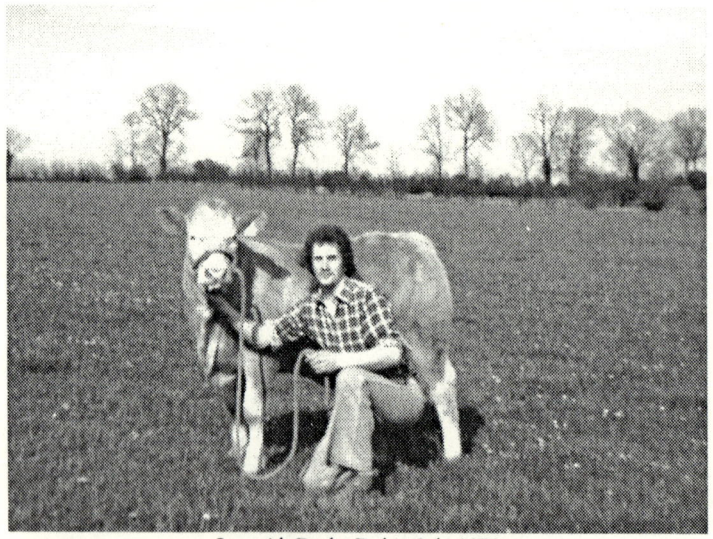

— *Ian with Derby Dyl in July 1979* —

Chapter Eleven
LIVESTOCK SHOWING

PRIOR TO THE ACCIDENT, MY BIG ENJOYMENT HAD BEEN showing beef cattle. In 1970, we had champion beast, a male with a twenty-two-month-old black Friesian-Angus cross named Sam. Sam was a beast that had suddenly improved his conformation and meat contents and so we decided to exhibit at a late date.

To gain champion status was a great surprise. We also took champion heifer (female) with a dark grey beast called Lulu. Preparing showing cattle takes a great deal of time, strength and patience. In those days I had plenty of time. In 1974, I lacked strength and my attitude towards killing livestock that I had gained trust with went against my feelings. I could not face the fact that to train animals for showing, you had to gain their trust and confidence so that you can lead them around the showroom. After all this, to then have the animal slaughtered just turned my stomach. During the years before my accident, we had grown from Christmas prime stock showing to competing in four summer shows. This was great fun. As my attitude had changed, I needed to find another category of livestock so that I required less strength and would not need to be too involved in gaining their trust.

I decided to go down the avenue of exhibiting lambs; these are sheep from birth till ten months old. These do not need so much strength and take less preparation for showing. The lambs do not need to be halter trained and do not need so much personal attention, and therefore I do not get too involved with the individual animals. We started showing at Christmas prime stock shows and gained a great deal of success. We then moved into summer shows for sheep classes.

At this time in 1976, my father's flock consisted of 150 female sheep. The ewes were mainly Suffolk-Mule cross. Within two years, I had increased the flock to 340 females. When we had lambed (sheep giving birth) the females we would result in a total of 600 to 640 lambs. Seventy of the 340 females would be lambed later in the first week of April, the others lambed mid-February. The reason we lambed the females later was so the lambs were not too large for the Christmas showing classes. This became full time planning and work. We had some good results at Rugby and Northampton Christmas shows.

The preparation of lambs for showing entails firstly making sure that the three animals to be shown as a group have identical meat content. This is judged by assessing the depth of their loin, the depth and length of the total body and a good content of meat on their rump. Fortunately, I have the gift for selecting lambs. In fact I became such an expert that I created a marketing group of my own that selected neighbouring farmers' lambs for slaughter. Sometimes the total of animals selected were six thousand per year. I enjoyed the organisation of the collection of these animals and payment of cheques. With my marketing of the lambs, this proved less time-consuming for the farmers, and a greater cheque total for the farmer. Also, this method of marketing sheep created less stress for the animals. This is beneficial for the welfare of the sheep. The direct transport of the lambs straight to the slaughterhouse creates a much more tender meat; also the direct transport saves much stress to the lamb.

Farmers would bring their lambs in their trailers and Land Rovers; the amount of lambs they brought to me was between six and forty lambs per trailer. The farmer had selected the lambs. The lambs would be herded into a pen which was a set size, and this would enable me to walk amongst them to select each lamb for slaughter. I would spray the initials of the farmer on the lamb's back. Each farmer had been given a colour code with his initial; this enables the slaughterhouse to identify the lambs when they arrive at the slaughterhouse.

A mass collection from my farm enabled me to transport them to the slaughterhouse at a cheaper rate. The brown transport lorry that arrived to collect the lambs of the day reversed up to the pens where the lambs were being held. Each farm's lambs were herded into the lorry and, when they had been penned with great care, a sectional door was closed to prevent them mixing with the other farmers' lambs. The pen that they were batched in within the lorry was large enough to stop overcrowding. This could result in

Livestock Showing

death or bruising of the flesh, which could devalue the meat. When the lambs arrived at the slaughterhouse, they were counted out of the lorry to make sure the invoice accompanying them had the right number written down. The initial on the lamb's back, which had been sprayed on by myself, was entered onto the slaughter sheet to enable prices to be paid to the correct farmer.

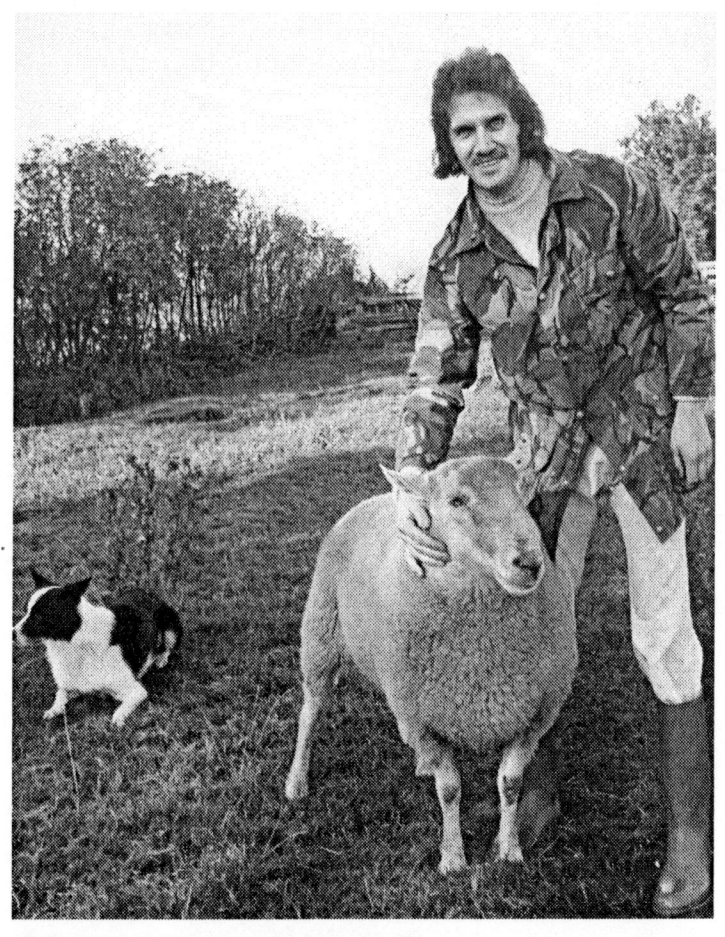

The farmer's selection at the beginning of my buying group was to be greatly improved within three months of commencing. The farmers, of mixed ages, were soon taught by me how to select lambs correctly. The lambs had to be selected for the modern meat requirements and also for the individual slaughterhouse classification. The lamb's weight and value were listed on the prices invoice with the farmer's name. The sheets arrived by post at my farm, three to four days after the slaughter. I then either faxed or phoned through the results to the farmers. The cheque for the value of the lambs was sent to me ten to fourteen days later; I divided the sum into the correct farmers' names and addresses and sent the farmers their cheques. All I used to charge was £1 per lamb commission: what cheap labour!

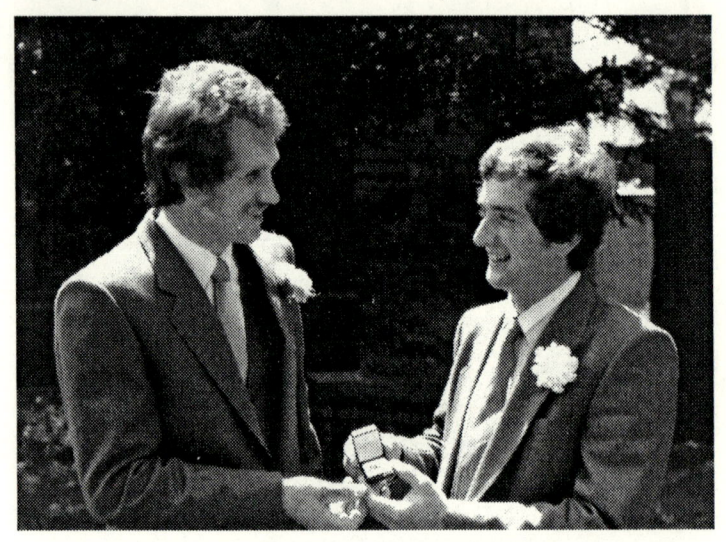

— *Ian with his best man, Russell Bailey, on his wedding day in June 1984* —

Chapter Twelve
BOWLS

IN MY YOUNGER DAYS, I HAD ENJOYED AND COMPETED HARD in rugby football. This was the only sport I enjoyed. Unfortunately now at my age and with my disabilities, rugby was a game that I could not take part in any more.

I decided to try and play lawn bowls at my nearby village in West Haddon. The bowls green was not a full size but it would start me on my new hobby. As I have mentioned, head-injury victims sometimes are poor on coordination and concentration; both of these I had difficulty with. My coordination was slowly improving; my concentration was something of a challenge. It was like a baby learning – but an oversized baby – and I was very aware of my coordination being poor. A bowls game consists of twenty-one 'ends'; this means that you go up and down the bowls green twenty-one times. You also have an extra two ends at the start of the game to get your weight and green in your mind. The equipment used for bowls is as follows: the player when competing in singles has four woods, which the player bowls on the green towards a white or yellow jack, and a rubber mat to stand on. The jack is delivered prior to each end that you play. The jack is placed at the length you bowl the jack and in the centre of the rink that you are playing on. Most bowls greens have six rinks. The idea of the game is for each player to try and get as near to the jack as possible.

After the first two ends of bowls my leg started to ache and my mind started to wander. At the halfway point of the game, my leg was giving me a lot of pain and my mind was still wandering. At the end of the game, my game was a mess – well, in my mind, anyway. I wanted near perfection. Dennis Orcherton, a player at West Haddon, was concerned about my lack of coordination and often visited my home and offered to chauffeur me anywhere. Thirty years on, I have not found perfection in my bowls game and that's after a great deal of effort, maybe too much effort and not relaxing enough. After my first three years competing at bowls for West Haddon, I had won two trophies, which I am very proud of.

The late Len Clark, a farmer from West Haddon, invited me to play for Rugby Bowling Club in the early 1980s. This club has its old tradition of inviting people to play for it. It is a well-known bowling club and produces a lot of good bowlers.

The green is full size and they play more games than West Haddon Club. West Haddon Club is a small club and does not have a set uniform to wear. The club also travels further to play bowls. The competition is greater at Rugby and you can be involved in many competition games. One of the most enjoyable parts in playing at Rugby is that you have to wear a set uniform, which looks very smart. In the mid-1980s I played a lot of bowls; it was a way of getting me out of the farming environment and away from the work I could not complete. I played one day in the week for West Haddon, one day for Rugby. Every other week, I would play for Rugby Bowling Association and occasionally I would play for Warwickshire Vice President's.

Taking part in bowls certainly helped me with my concentration and coordination, although it made me very tired at the start of my new hobby. In fact it made me tired for twenty-five years. The reason was that the flat shoes you wear for bowls stretched my left leg guide more than it was used to when wearing proper shoes with heels. But I would advise anybody suffering similarly to myself either from an accident or a stroke to take part in lawn bowls as it is good exercise. It involves you with other people, young and old, male and female. Players are always welcome at any bowls club. The social life is very good.

Bowls

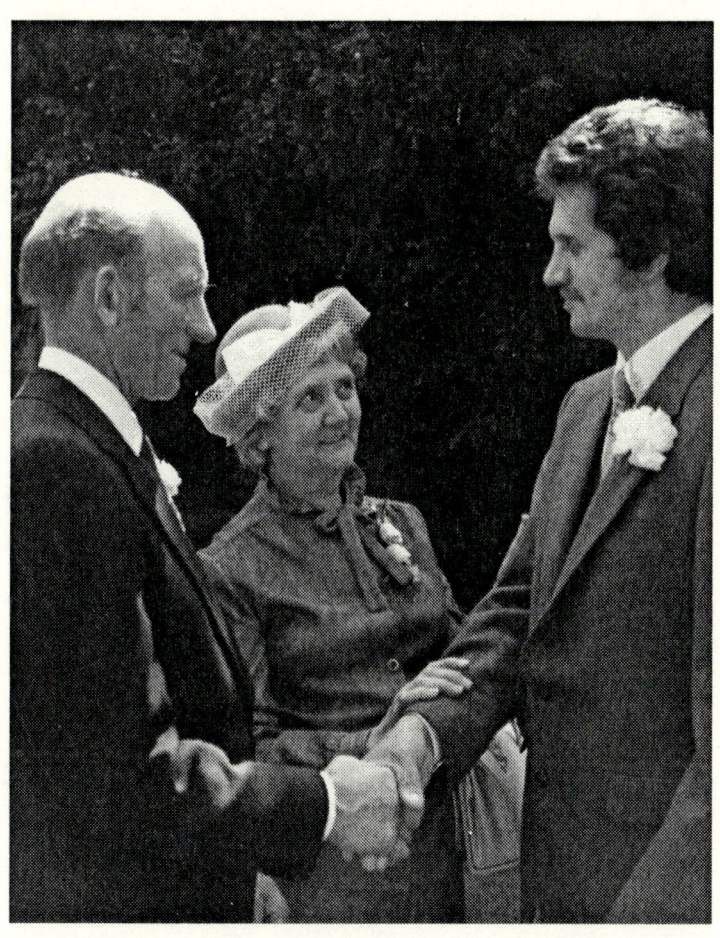

— *Ian's wedding, June 1984. Father, Mother and Ian* —

Chapter Thirteen
JUST WORK

MY FATHER, LIKE MOST FARMERS OF HIS GENERATION, worked seven days a week and hardly ever took a day off or a holiday. His weekly or fortnightly outing to market to sell or purchase his cattle or sheep, which would either be to Rugby or Northampton, was his only time out. It is quite funny, really; I have only just realised that I was robbing Father of his infrequent social outings. My father was five feet nine inches and bald. He had been bald since the age of twenty after a lime bag fell on him and some of the lime went over his head and shoulders, hence stopping his hair growth. He seldom smiled but when he did it made me feel more relaxed. He had always been slim and fit. He was not an outgoing sort of person. As I started taking more interest in the farm, and especially the sheep sales, he used to stop at home working, often only going to special cattle sales. Father had a love for cattle. He always attended the annual prime stock shows at Christmas, as he had a great interest in either cattle we were exhibiting or the lambs. These outings and work on the farm were really his two delights, which I am pleased to say we enjoyed together.

After the disappointment of leaving my employment in Daventry Farm Shop (the Farm Shop was a dark green wooden framed window in a brick building which had an upper and lower level, situated in the middle of Daventry), I decided the way forward was to take up swimming. Swimming was embarrassing for me, as my left foot continuously dragged along the floor. My left shoe's toe leather wore away very quickly. Also the lack of movement of my hip had caused an excess of flesh on my left side. Often I wished I could cut this flesh off with a knife and feed it to the dogs. Hence I decided to work with my father to help my fitness, and really that was the only job I could do.

Gosh, it was hard work, and very tiring! I never liked to have any challenge beat me – the times we have worked for five hours in the morning, stopped for one hour at lunchtime and then commenced a further four hours' work. At this time it was very difficult for me to catch a sheep. As my coordination was awfully slow, I would go to move one way and the sheep would be three yards away in the next second: highly embarrassing, and again I felt like a child. I often imagined the sheep laughing at me as they ran away. Father never laughed but always used to say, 'There will be another time.' But I'm damned if I have ever experienced this in the first twenty-nine years of my recovery!

My leg would become so heavy; I treated it like another person. I called him 'Ned'. Often Ned and I would have a disagreement about what to do next, or if he wanted to go bowling. Ned partly won the battle. Firstly, he was too tired to go out at night. This argument he won for two years. The other complaint, he often used to win, is if he felt so unsightly and did not want or need to be seen, either limping up the bowls green or in a pair of swimming trunks; in fact he stopped going swimming because he found his leg and his figure too embarrassing. He felt perfection or near perfection was needed to be viewed by other people. He still thinks, thirty years on and now knocking on fifty years old, that his leg is a total embarrassment wherever he goes.

My leg used to ache from 11 a.m. to 6 p.m. Once I sat down the pain stopped. I am lucky – the pain eventually went. Something many people have to suffer is endless pain with their legs or limbs and this is very tiring. The pain in my legs lasted until 1982, seven days a week, partly because I pushed myself further each day in the hope of total recovery. I decided to ease off with the heavy and continuous work; as I did this the pain decreased. As I was working seven days a week, Sundays became my relaxing day. I would go shepherding. Shepherding is when you go around the sheep and cattle in the field and checking that they are all present and also that they have no health problems such as sore feet; in the summer their eyes could become watery with the effects of sun and they would not be looking sick. A sheep that looks sick would have its ears flat rather than erect. It would be standing on its own and looking totally uncomfortable

Just Work

and empty. I would then call round to elderly friends for a coffee or tea. This for two years was my only contact with people other than my family, as I was intent working myself back to health.

For six years I concentrated on my work with the sheep and I also went green bowling. Bowling starts usually the last week in April and finishes the last week in September. Unfortunately, as I improved my bowls I became more involved in the farm. Quite often I would have to phone my club and pull out of the team. Sometimes this was only three days before the match; my team and club mates didn't appreciate how busy farm life could be. In June I might have to withdraw from the game because the hay would be fit for baling on the Saturday, and Saturday was the weekend games of bowls; if the hay was not baled when it was fit it would lose its feeding value when it was fed to the cattle and sheep in the winter months. Although I was mainly involved in livestock farming, I liked the challenge of helping my brother move the corn from the field to the grain store.

This involved driving a tractor, which towed a trailer from which we offloaded corn in the field, and it was a great challenge to reach the corn store and be back in the field to collect the next tank of corn. The tank on the combine held approximately a ton and a half of corn; the trailer with five foot deep sides held approximately four tons of corn.

Another upset to my bowls days would be when we were still lambing the sheep during the third week in April. I was in charge of the lambing sheep. We lambed in April, as we took part in Christmas shows with the lambs. If the lambs were born earlier than April than they would have been too heavy for the classes. I will tell you about the detail planning of the sheep later. All the timing of the harvest, haying and lambing was very important. If the corn was fit and not harvested at the right time it could either get too dry and shrivel and fall out of the corn head; or if it rained the corn would go mouldy. Here was another instance where if I played bowls we might lose the value of the corn completely.

As I promised earlier on, I will explain why I had to be present when my sheep were lambing. At the birth if the lambs were presented incorrectly, such as one leg back or coming out backwards, it would be impossible for the ewe (female sheep) to give birth, that is why my being present was very important. If I hadn't been there it would have meant great pain, possible loss of life, and loss of money. I seldom asked anybody except my father to look after the sheep because I was very particular about the care of my sheep. Father was as competent as I was, so I did not have to worry if I asked him to look after the sheep. Like anything I do, I put a lot of time and thought into it. If my father was unavailable to help I could not have afforded to find somebody good enough; plus I liked the challenge of husbandry, of looking after my flock. Sometimes one's work has to take place of one's sport.

Chapter Fourteen
SECURITY LIFE

THE YEAR 1998 WAS A BAD ONE FOR ME. WE HAD JUST dissolved the farming partnership between my father, Phillip and myself. Fortunately enough we farmed three farms that were fairly close together. My brother farmed and lived on the Grange Farm in West Haddon parish. He also farmed seventy-two acres called The Covert Farm, situated on the A5 just north of Junction 18 of the M1. My share of the partnership was the Wold Farm in Crick parish, on the West Haddon road between Crick and West Haddon. My parents lived on this farm, and I lived in a small bungalow in Crick, which was a mile and a half from the Wold Farm. Phillip had always preferred the arable side of farming – that is, cultivation of the ground for various crops. I always preferred the livestock side of farming, which meant I needed a lot of grass fields to feed my sheep and cattle. There is one drawback with livestock: you have to be very physically fit and it involved a lot of lifting and pulling every day.

My back had been weak from the first year of the accident but this year it had become a lot worse. It was so fragile when being amongst the sheep; one small knock and I suffered severe pain. Also, trying to restrain a sheep caused great damage to my back. This meant I had to employ more labour to help with the flock of sheep, somebody to turn them over so I could trim their feet. I also needed someone to catch them so I could trim their rear end; this is called 'dagging'. All these expenses became too much for the farm to make a profit; the bills were eating into the previous year's profit. I had got to do something to make things work better. Much against my father's wishes – although not a financial partner, I did not like to change the way my father had farmed for years – I decided to change the method rather than be in great financial distress.

After many months of thought in ways I could change the method of farming, I thought the easiest way ahead was to rent thirty-six acres of grass for the period 1 April to 30 October to a farming neighbour. Father was not amused; but it had to be done to make the farm break even. I decided to sell 150 ewes – female sheep. These I would have normally lambed in January to February. I sold these in August and September so as to enable other farmers to buy so that they could lamb them in 1999. A ewe's pregnancy is one 143 days to one 148.

With more time to spare, I decided to look for a job to bring some money in. I had no qualifications for office work, and being shut in a room would have been quite boring, but one has to take what one can get. I needed a job where I would be appreciated and possibly where I would be meeting many people. I decided to apply for a security vacancy at Eddie Stobart's, at Crick DIRFT Estate. Crick DIRFT site is situated in 170 acres of land, north-west of Junction 18, virtually between the A5 link road and the M1. The job that I applied for was a gatehouse officer. I was given the job as all it required was a smart trustworthy person who could cope with phone work and signing lorries in and out.

On the first evening, as I was working from 6 p.m., I was instructed to be at the gatehouse at 5 p.m. to receive instructions for my work to be carried out. Well, by 6 p.m. no one arrived to show me how to proceed. Luckily enough I had been watching the officer on the day shift; when he finished his shift I took over. Well, it was just like arrows being shot at me by a group of bowmen. They say practice makes perfect. By the time I finished my shift at 6 a.m., I was seeing lorries in every direction, in my dreams and in my office. This job unfortunately only lasted ten weeks, as my father passed away very suddenly, which meant that I had to forego the job and return to manage the farm, as we were soon to be into the lambing season.

I loved going off on my own little ventures without telling a soul, especially when looking for a job vacancy. After all I was over twenty-one! One day before I was to start my job at Eddie Stobart's I was having a heated discussion with Father. He had accepted the land being rented out and could the see the benefit to the farm. The only way of making a living for me was not to undertake too much lifting and pulling, which is continually involved in sheep farming. Father accepted I could not do too much sheep handling work but thought that I would be content with the ninety ewes that I had remaining to lamb in January 1999. How wrong – I need money and a challenge. The main content of the heated argument was that I had no qualifications to find a job, which would bring in enough money.

'Well,' I said, 'I have found a job and I start tomorrow.'

There was a silence for a minute or two. Father then said, 'If you have found a job you can cope with and will bring in enough money for you, I do not blame you; it will pay you better than farming.'

Little did he know I was only working three twelve-hour shifts, but the money these earned me was more than the farm would earn in three weeks.

Ned

I need to tell a story
About Ned
He struggled to cope
From day to day
He would not go out.
If he did go out he felt inferior
To all those he met
He hid if he could
Stood pain when he stood
He asked for no consideration
He is getting old
Do you think you know
Who could it be?
It is my slow old leg...
Ned.

Home
12 June 2002

Rugby Advertiser Article, 1979
INJURIES CHANGED STUDENT'S LIFE

A Farmer's son, Ian Litchfield, had been a student at an agricultural college and a keen rugby player when in March 1972, when he was 18, he was involved in an accident which left him with brain damage. Ian, now 25, of Grange Farm, West Haddon, has had to give up his studies and his sport.

He had been a passenger in a van and was thrown out, after being in collision with another van, sustaining serious head-injuries.

Ian said he planned to write a book about his experience 'to help others who have suffered brain damage in an accident'.

He said he would not go back to college but still hoped to stay in farming.

Ian played rugby for a local village team and had trials with the All-England Young Farmers XV.

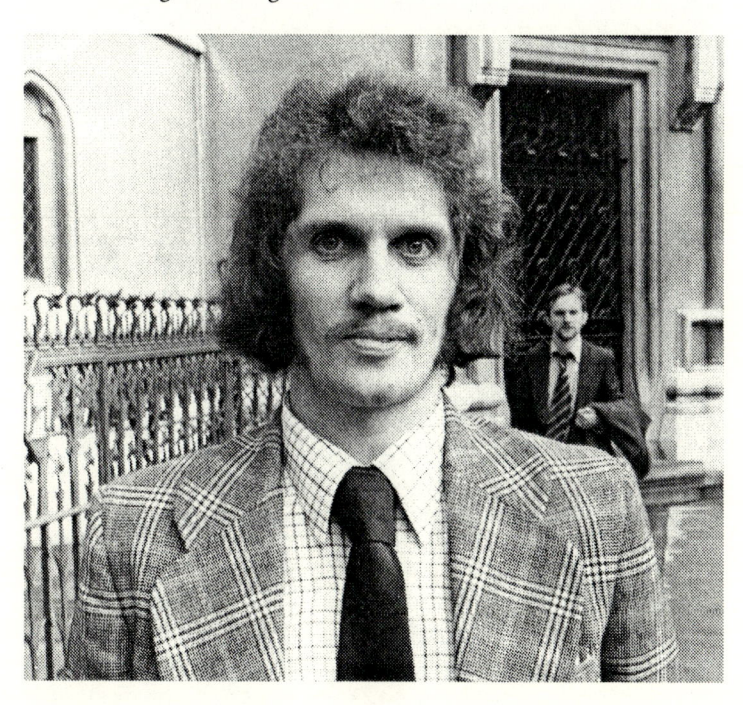

Chapter Fifteen
REFLECTIONS

IN THE FIRST STAGES OF RECOVERING AFTER RETURNING home from hospital I tried too hard. I did not, at times, have the patience or understanding to pace myself. How was I going to cope with everyday life, never mind keeping up with Father with his farm work and achievements?

It was as if I was in my own world. It is hard to explain to someone how it feels for me to see people my own age running about; that is something that still is so annoying. I am a mature man; I have not been able to run for thirty years. It might be strange for you to understand but it makes me feel so pathetic and inept.

A thing that has not improved is carrying a glass or cup full of liquid. It doesn't matter which hand I use. The damage sustained by the right side of my brain in the accident affects the left side of my body. I can not carry one glass without spilling it. I have found the only way to conquer this task is to have two or three sips before I start to move. People's looks when I have moved like an old snail crossing a room, still managing to spill the drink! They must be thinking, *Pathetic*, or *Good God, he's drunk*! Maybe these thoughts were only in my head. But still to this day if I believe somebody is looking at me I tend to spill the drink or start to limp. It is all a matter of nerves, I think. Aged forty-eight and I cannot carry a drink. Oh, how embarrassing and pathetic...

My speech has improved tremendously but still gets a little confused with my brain. If I try to talk as fast as I think, I get the same old troubles, my brain works faster than my speech and my body. This is the world I live in; I suspect I am not the only one. I would love to compare my world and experiences with other people involved with head-injuries.

One thing which is understandable, because people do not realise, is that friends or parents of the victim can be too quick in coming to the aid of the person. At certain times you need some help, but please give us self-respect and let us help ourselves. It is in our best interests. How often I would go to bed at night feeling shattered. I'd be pleased at what I had achieved, but thinking if only there was a life where you did not have to keep experiencing pain and working hard just to keep up with other people so as to keep your self-respect.

It would be nice to have a straight arm and two strong legs. In the early stages of my recovery I named my left leg 'Ned'. Every day, every time I walk I have to think about making sure my knee did not 'back knee'. My toes and ankle, which fail to move, and my calf muscle, are not strong enough to support the action of my knee. This puts more pressure on the knee, causing me to limp more. It's frustrating, after thirty years.

Well, I think and hope I have given a reasonable description of 'Another World' that many of us live in, and few have expressed how they feel. I do hope this will give victims of injury or a stroke a lot of help. Parents and relatives will read this and hopefully if involved in such incidents will have some understanding about how to cope with the victim. The victim is going through such a frustrating time meeting the great challenges every day; this varies between individual head accidents.

In the first three years I suffered long deep depressions, sometimes lasting six to eight weeks. One of the occasions I often look back on was a wonderful game of rugby I played in 1971 for Long Buckby second team. I travelled to Wellingborough in the team's coach. Tea was served, and entertainment was provided in the form of a disco. Although I was young and innocent this did not stop me viewing and dancing with the young ladies. I had just sat down after dancing to the Rolling Stones' *I Can't Get No Satisfaction* when a young lady asked me if I could help her start her car. The lady's name was Jade. She had long dark straight hair, I think green eyes, and a voluptuous figure. Jade's hair looked darker as she had a pale complexion.

Not wanting to tell her I knew little about engines, her stunning figure in her very fitted dress persuaded me to go and look at the car. The car park was situated at the side of the clubhouse, with bushes and trees surrounding on three sides. Jade's car was at the rear of the car park. She took me by the hand as we left the clubhouse and showed me where the car was parked. She led me past her car into the bushes. It was then that she admitted her car was fine. She had seen me in the clubhouse and fancied me. The next thing, she pulled me on to the ground. I was taken by great surprise and did not resist.

Well, I landed smack onto her lovely breasts; it was just as if I was on the sea but maybe a little softer. Jade said, 'I want you to service my engine.' Now, being an innocent young gentleman, I thought it was rude to disappoint her. Your imagination can take over from here. I did raise a few important items with her.

David Evans, who was one of my team players in the second team, was, with Bill Mawby, in charge of the players on the coach. They looked everywhere for me, as the remainder wanted to go home. The coach eventually left for the home destination.

When Jade, who by now was feeling tired, and I, who was feeling the effects of the last-minute exercise, appeared one and a half hours after entering the bushes, we found my transport had gone.

Jade made a hard deal with me. If she was to take me home in her car she expected me to come and service her engine. She decided that my attention to detail was preferred to her present mechanic, who serviced her quite regularly. For three weeks she required my attention. This I agreed to. Up until this date my team-mates did not know how I got home earlier than they did, even though I started back later than they did.

These rugger memories often used to be relived in my head. It made me feel like an old man with few capabilities, just like a child trying to learn new tricks.

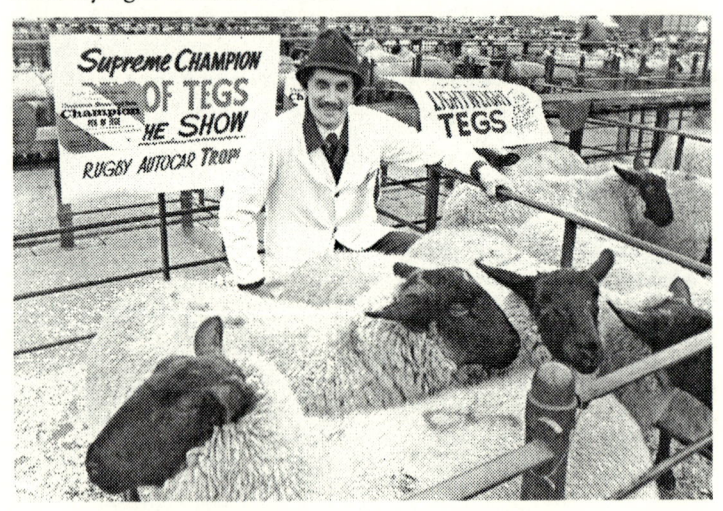

— *Champion Lambs at Rugby Market 1976* —

Chapter Sixteen
FEBRUARY

IN FEBRUARY 2001 I WAS EMPLOYED AT MALCOLM'S TRANSPORT Distribution Company at DIRFT in Crick. Yes, still at DIRFT, next door to my last security position at Tibbett and Britten, also a distribution company.

I made my regular physio visit and this regular outing was causing me great concern. In my mind, having my bones pushed back each time must be wearing them down. The chiropractic manipulator, Gus Gibbon, lived at Church Lawford, which is four miles Coventry side of Rugby and nine miles from my home in Crick.

On this visit Gus was having a trial period with a new device called PAM (Power-Assisted Micro Manipulator). This machine was invented by Robert Taylor. The first chance to use this machine was in 2000 and it is still being trialled.

This device was circular in shape with a combination of vibrating metal balls. This is moved lightly over the area of the body which is either lacking muscle or suffering severe pain or is lacking movement.

The next three weeks I could not believe the pain I was feeling in my left thigh. The PAM device had encouraged my muscles to work for the first time in twenty-nine years: tear-jerking for me.

In February I noticed an advert in our local newspaper: *Acupuncture – a free session*. That sounded interesting and free. With nothing to lose, I made my appointment. I visited the acupuncture room, which was at a dental surgery at Bilton. Bilton is a village which neighbours Rugby on the Coventry side.

The dental surgery was a dark wooden-built building with large paned windows. As I entered the dental surgery I was met by a glowing young lady. Gosh, she was gorgeous, with shoulder-length dark hair; she also had stunning eyes. She was five feet six inches tall with a fantastic figure, and her name was Mandi.

February

Mandi was the receptionist and she asked me to take a seat. I said, 'Where to?'

Mr Jose Lacey, the acupuncturist, welcomed me into his room. I was asked a lot of questions concerning my health condition, and he asked if I was on any medication, which I wasn't, and what I hoped to improve with the treatment.

I was then asked to lie on the couch with my sleeves rolled up and my trousers left on his chair. Pins were placed in areas of concern, left temple, left elbow, my left knee and ankle. I remained with these pins in my body for I think fifteen minutes. I asked once to move and have one pin in my ankle replaced, as it was not very comfortable. I must say I was thinking when I had my next drink the fluid might run out of the pin holes! Sorry, I could not resist that little quip.

I visited Mr Lacey twice a month, and then once a month for two months, and now every six weeks.

I just could not believe it. My ankle actually started to move for the first time in thirty years. This was quite unbelievable.

Could I have had more mobility if I had the acupuncture earlier on? Or was it a matter of time healing the damage caused in the accident?

One morning I decided to gather the remaining sheep that I had kept when I'd sold the others the previous September. Eighteen was the total number of sheep left. The reason for collecting the sheep was to check their feet. Well, the sheep must have thought, *Here comes handicap Sam*. The sheep knew that in the past years they had always been able to outmanoeuvre me. One ewe made a break for it; I suddenly broke into a run and caught the old devil. I do not know who was the most surprised. The ewe... her eyes looked a mist of shock! I just stood there and thought, *Bloody hell, I can run after thirty years*! I shook with emotions, my eyes were filling with water, and I just broke into tears. I am back in your world now, able to run at last.

It was so ruddy emotional I think it was better than sex; sex you can repeat but this marvellous achievement hopefully would remain.

Physiotherapy and gym work had a lot to play in my recovery. Physio for the last eight months has been with John Gratham at

Long Buckby village in his house. He had and is still concentrating on building strength into my left leg. My left leg is now becoming similar to my right. Gym work has been only going on for the last five weeks. I have not been in the pool yet because of the disgusting unsightly extra flesh in my left side. Since my left leg has been functioning better, this causes less pain in my knee and more pain in my left side, as it causes muscles that have not moved for thirty years to work again.

Gosh, is the body not a wonderful creation! I hope by autumn the extra flesh will have vanished away with exercise. I hope I'll be able to walk almost correctly.

Since all these things started to happen in February, I have been walking around with tears in my eyes, pleased to be back in your world, able to go swimming and look respectable and not appear like a leper when walking along the streets or down the bowling green. I feel as if I have been born again. Life really has been worth all the effort. All the pain and frustration has been justified.

Life

Have a good time
I always did and you always will
Life is for living. Life is short.
Many people cannot walk or talk
So why should we complain
We are all part of life in this world
Part of the big game
When we die the world will live on
No matter what we say
The world will go on
Just enjoy and savour every minute
Of every day
Thank you all for your patience.

Home
7 June 2002

Chapter Seventeen
EMOTIONS

MY FAMILY LIFE HAS ALWAYS BEEN HARD WORK. FATHER AND Mother are rarely to be seen out together. Father always prefers to stop at the farm working. His generation, born in the mid-1920s, were always working to earn a living.

My mother was the one who had to take my brother and me out for a treat. Father was a withdrawn person and very shy. He lived for work, not worked to live. He was a person who, in his whole life, never showed any loving emotions towards me; but we respected each other without even saying so.

Until after the accident I had not thought about emotions. After the accident I had long periods of depression. I hated myself. I felt a total disgrace to my parents. In the first two years I was virtually unmanageable with my parents and nurses. With people I did not know before the accident I was okay.

I was interested in girls and had always found them appealing and very knowledgeable, and always a tremendous challenge. I had various girlfriends but found no lasting emotions, and at the age of thirty I wondered if I would ever get married.

In 1984, when I was thirty-four, I got married to a lady called Dilys – a fine Welsh name. After this event I improved tremendously. But as I improved in health, my emotions, of which I had few, seemed to die.

I separated from my wife in November 1995. We had grown apart and did not want to live in a speechless and emotionless marriage. The day I left my wife I asked her to pack my bags for me and I wrote her a letter saying she could have the car and the house, but nothing else, except the furniture she owned.

I stopped at a friend's hotel at West Haddon. I stayed in the wooden staff bungalow which was divided into three. My room's furniture consisted of one bed, one television and one toilet (real modern stuff).

In 1996, I met a lady with short dark hair; she was five feet eight inches and walked with an authoritative step. This person does not want to be named. I had respect for this lady, she had high standards and was a great help to me. I know this person helped me to relax and start to gain respect for myself. As I have mentioned, my driving capabilities were crap. She would drive me everywhere I wanted to go without complaining. In the early years she was not working and she always hoped I would pay for the fuel, which I was only too eager to do.

Seven years on it was happening again; we had grown apart. We both had our own interests and lives to follow. As I already described, I had lost the ability to show any lasting emotion in a relationship. Everything I took on was a tremendous challenge.

On 28 April 2002 we decided to part. We had parted company before but got together again. I very much hope that this lady finds a man who can give her what she deserves in the way of a happy and sociable life.

The following Friday, in Crick post office, I was collecting an evening paper for my mother. The post office is full of stock and there's not a great deal of space for people to walk around the shop. This was a good thing on this occasion. As I gently moved towards a gorgeous young lady, I would say about five feet seven inches, with long dark hair and a tanned complexion, I heard her ask a lady there if she knew of anybody who required someone to type. This was fate, as I was looking for a person to help type this book.

I excused myself to her and mentioned I had overhead her enquiry about a typing job.

I had never felt this way before; I had seen her infectious smile, heard her wonderful accent – not being sure what accent it was. She was dressed in a black leather coat with a nicely fitted black dress. I later found out, as you would say in farming terms, that she was a 'Scottish-Irish cross'.

I, for the first time, had fallen in love. Emotions I feared I did not have flowed. I gave her my phone number, scribbled on the back of a fuel receipt. I told her if she was interested in a short-term job to contact me. I did not ask her name, as I believed for the first time in my life I was speechless – very unusual for me.

Three days passed, and I felt confused about my feelings. I never had eyes feeling so painful with the pressure of tears behind them. I continually felt I was going to break down and cry. For thirty years I found I had no lasting emotions. But could this be the start of a new experience.

The lady in the shop did not phone me for one week. When she did phone me she told me her name was Becky. She showed great interest when I told her about the book I was writing. When we met the next day, it was as if the world had stopped. She was the first person who I thought I could love, though I had decided this event was never to be.

Becky came to my home twice to discuss the book, and we both found ourselves relaxed in each other's company. When leaving my bungalow on the second occasion, going out of the large hallway, Becky turned around. She looked into my eyes – she looked stunning – she was wearing a light brown trouser suit and had a wonderful smile. Our eyes met. She had told me she was twenty-six – twenty-seven on 17 June. She was separated. We slowly moved towards each other. I reached out with my right hand and tenderly took hold of her left hand, as our bodies touched I gently kiss her forehead and her left ear.

Becky responded gently, snuggling into my chest. As she came closer I could not hold back my tears any longer; they rolled on to Becky's beautiful smiling cheeks. Becky quietly said, 'I thought it would be years before I met somebody I could love and care for.'

Becky said, 'I would like to get to know you and all your friends and learn your lifestyle.'

'Gosh,' I said, 'how can a beautiful young lady like you want to get involved with an old man like me – especially with my goofy leg and arm?'

Becky quietly replied, 'Age is something that we can cope with, as I hope we will learn to respect and love each other, but we must not rush into these things, as I do not want to get hurt again.'

I had, by now, pulled my emotions together and stopped crying, and I replied, 'If there is any chance of you and I becoming involved, I have no intentions of rushing. Your company is something I would greatly respect.'

For the first time in my life I had no fear of being totally involved with someone. I was smitten. As my driving capabilities were still very poor it was nice to hear that she only lived four miles away in the town of Rugby.

Ladies

All my life I have made time for ladies
They will make time to talk and discuss
And listen to all my plans
And help me if they can.

Hazel was my first girlfriend when I was ten
To church I went to complete my plan
Carol was next – such a dark-haired delight.

Kathryn was there to comfort me
Rachel gave help with my livestock plan
Jill was always ready to give me a hand
Night or day, Ann was a delight – but always at work
Carol, who I lost touch with, I would love to meet again.

Ruth was fantastic but wanted to marry
I was not ready, so declined with frustration
Dilys was next, I think,
It all got rather hazy when I was thirty-six
Marriage lasted a few years but flowed down the river
Another lady was there to give such care
At last a fantastic lady that I could give some care.

Seven years passed and I was off again
To new pastures to make hay again
Will I ever learn, or am I such a pain?
God, what a shame!

Chapter Eighteen
DRIVING

AFTER THE ACCIDENT I WAS NOT ALLOWED TO DRIVE FOR three years. Once I was allowed to drive it gave me a much more independent life.

It was after one of my regular examinations they found that my eyes required glasses for a distance correction. It was like, I think, heaven to take myself out to see friends, or take somebody out for the evening.

Mother encountered tremendous nervous problems. The doctor who gave me the go ahead for driving told me to make short journeys provisionally as my brain and eyesight would need some time to adjust to the new stress and learning process.

Mother faced a great void after me regaining my independence through driving, and worried that whilst driving my brain might find it too much and relapse, causing me to have an accident. The often daily routine of taking me out in the afternoon – as I needed the break – had gone, and also the trip out that my mother very much needed after the tremendous difficulties she had experienced with my long depressions and bloody-mindedness, together with my attitude of not accepting any physical help.

When I was driving myself out Mother always wanted to know where I was going and what time I would be back; it made me feel such a child. Only after did I realise how worrying it must have been. My coordination still needed to be greatly improved. Here is how I would cope with this. If I knew when I was driving out, on that day I would not be involved with heavy, physical work, as the effect of this on my body was that it would take my left foot ten minutes to decide where it was going, and my left arm would become very bent. I can see the funny side now as I write this, but at the time it was a continual trouble to me and a mind-boggling affair for my parents to deal with.

Driving

After a few months, the continuous driving, which helped me get away from work I could not cope with, started to give me double vision and bad headaches. I did not complain but slowly found reasons to explain why I would not visit some people, if they were more than fifteen miles away. I decided that it was far more important to cope with the manual labour and improve my fitness than it was to drive to a lot of places.

I used to accept, in the first ten years, the fact that I could not cope with driving further than fifteen miles at one time. Friends were very understanding. Once I got past the ten years mark, I found it very embarrassing to ask anybody to drive me to various places. I did not ask people to go out of their way, but to take me to the venue if they were going. I think some people used to think I was too tight-fisted in not using my car and petrol. As years went by it became more and more embarrassing to admit that my head was unable to cope with the stress and concentration of driving.

As the years went past, driving became more stressful for everybody. I think it has certainly become more difficult for myself to accept my lack of driving capabilities.

I often used to get depressed with my leg and arm looking unsightly and feeling very tired. Then, to find I could not take myself away from hard labour became very hurtful and embarrassing. This was something else I had not realised would be the case. To ask for a ride from someone was so degrading and that has not improved (God, I do sound ungrateful!). It's so embarrassing to admit again that I am restricted like a child.

The accident I was involved in has not given me any phobia against either my driving capabilities or as a passenger. I was not driving either of the two vehicles involved in my accident. Most of the people who have driven me place to place have been very good drivers; any driver I did not feel safe with I always found some reason not to ride with again.

The lady who helped me regain my respect and my social contacts and initially to regain my life was a tremendous driver. Her limitations were none (we are talking about driving). If, when en route to a farm to either select lambs for marketing or to purchase a new ram (male sheep), we took the wrong route she

Driving

never got flustered; she would just turn the car around and try again. So nice! (God, how I miss that comforting hug and that tremendous kiss – but life must go on.)

What I found easiest to drive was the Land Rover, which is a four-wheel drive vehicle. Possibly this was due to the fact that it was not as fast as a car, and the movement of fast-moving vehicles did confuse my brain or my eyesight. I found I could drive further using the Land Rover than if I was driving another car. Also, when driving the Land Rover I was sat a lot higher in the vehicle, which gives you a far better view of the oncoming traffic.

I decided three years ago to sell my Vauxhall Corsa and also my Land Rover. In place of these I bought a Daihatsu Fourtrack vehicle. This was a far more presentable vehicle when socialising, but also had the four-wheel drive capability for my farm work.

Chapter Nineteen
RUTH

'IN MY EXPERIENCE OF THIRTY YEARS OF TRAUMA AND orthopaedic nursing, Ian has made the most complete recovery from a severe head-injury that I have witnessed. This is all due to his bloody-minded determination. I always believed he would do it. As I am speaking to him now, I realise this recovery has entered a new phase.'

Ruth remembers the day I was admitted to the George and Elizabeth wards from the emergency and accident section. There were two similar victims on that day. Ruth remembers it particularly well, as it was quite early for a student nurse to be involved not with one patient but two. To her, they both looked fit, well-muscled young men with no damage to their body. Their heads were the only parts damaged. Ruth had to look after me, as the senior nurse was in control of the other victim. Both of the patients were put in a two-bed section. This section had a sliding partition, which enabled the senior nurse to slide the section back so she could oversee the treatment Ruth was giving.

Both of us eventually suffered bleeding into the brain requiring burr holes drilled into the skull to relieve the pressure on the brain. The chance of our survival was ninety to ten against. The hospital was preparing the theatres for the operations. Mr Scott Ferguson was the surgeon on duty.

I remained in the Intensive Treatment Unit for four weeks. Ruth was on duty in the George and Elizabeth wards; she often used to visit the ITU and see my condition.

Only as I write this book and I am sitting in Ruth's home (by the way, she is still gorgeous) have I been told by her that after such a serious operation they give you three tests on the brain, ten days after the operation.

The first two tests were negative. Three different doctors

conduct these tests. The outlook was quite grim. The third test showed slight brain activity; if there had been no sign of life, the ventilator, which was keeping me alive, would have been switched off. Unfortunately, the other patient did not survive the operation.

To help me take nourishment, four days after the accident I was fitted with a tracheotomy – this is a plastic socket that was fitted into my throat, and a pipe was then fitted into the socket to enable me to be fed liquid food or special food prepared for me. I was unable to feed myself for the first seven weeks after my accident.

Ruth and I seemed to understand from our second meeting that I was determined to return to my able body, never mind what I had to do.

As I have mentioned, I could not feed myself and I hated people trying to help me. I was very stroppy and if I could not cope – stand back! – as I was seen to throw plates of food, cups, anything I could grab with my able right hand.

I did not like being dressed by anybody. I would get my good arm in the sleeve but could not get my left arm in. Often I got frustrated and lost patience, and the garment that I was trying to put on would end up being thrown across the other side of the ward or stuffed to the bottom of my bed. Or I would completely lose my control and flop down in the chair. At this time my coordination and balance were completely like a new-born baby.

If the nurses bed bathed me and cleaned my head, as I had no hair, and then dressed me, within thirty minutes I was in a mess, a real mess. If I tried to eat a meal, three quarters would land on my clothes and the other on the floor. If they had sat me out of bed in a chair, I quite often would fall out. Nobody could touch me, otherwise I would scream out. Maybe I might try to walk and would fall over; I would then crawl along the floor to the bed and try and walk again. Oops, there I go on the floor again... Often Ruth would find me on the floor in a heap. In a jovial way she would say, 'What on earth are you doing down there again, are you hiding from somebody? Well, it is about time you got up, we both know you can.'

We both had the same impression that I could do it eventually if I took on the challenge. Ruth knew how to handle me – that sounds good, doesn't it?

Mother had a fear of me falling and hurting myself. All mothers hold a fear for their children. In my case it was for my best interest to keep attempting things that I could not cope with.

Ruth says that she would often leave me for ten minutes and say, 'It is about time you could do this particular job.' When she returned I was either in a mess with food all over me or I was in a huddle on the floor with that silly grin.

Two years after I left Northampton Hospital I visited Ruth at her home in Northampton. Unfortunately, the promise that we had agreed on, which was for me to be at Ruth's twenty-first birthday, I could not keep, due to being at Rivermead Hospital. When she met me on her driveway in front of her house I put my arms around her waist and lifted her in a half-turn. This was so emotional for Ruth and me. It meant I had developed my strength back and could lift her. We both had tears in our eyes; it was a tremendous recovery in such a short time. This was as good a feeling as it would have been dancing with Ruth at her twenty-first birthday party, which I could not attend.

Chapter Twenty
LAST CHAPTER

MY BODY, ONCE UNSIGHTLY AND WITH LACK OF CO-ordination, is returning to near fitness. Meeting Becky and my sudden recovery all happened as I was trying to write *Another World*. The resulting feeling was, I do believe, like being in heaven. As I have always been rather spontaneous, I have made a sudden decision to play in my retirement game of rugby at Long Buckby. I cannot report the full outcome of my plans to play three games of rugby: one at Long Buckby, one at Northampton Town – I hope to have my name included on the Saints Rugby Team – and also my everlasting wish to have my name included with the England Rugby Team for the start of an international game.

The goal that I set myself in 1972 to play rugby again has started to look far from possible. I could not even run and my right temple was very tender even to touch. Also I was growing older. On 1 May 2002 I decided to visit David Evans who lived on a farm on the gated road between West Haddon and Long Buckby. He played rugby in the late 1960s with myself. We both played for Long Buckby first team – what memories! I wanted to tell him of my recent improvements to my left ankle and my complete left side. He and his wife, Joy, were overjoyed to hear the news; they thought it was a miracle. I also wanted to ask David about the possibility of playing in the three rugby games that I mentioned in the last paragraph. If you do not set yourself a goal your achievements will never be as high.

David said, 'Nothing is impossible, leave it to me.' I guess it's all down to what each person needs to achieve. The accident on 16 March 1972 seems to have made me feel so inferior to everybody else and to need to prove myself in everything I do. I hope that if I can complete my rugby ambitions, and if Becky is given time to understand me and my life, as I am always out to achieve, I think with Becky by my side, in my bed, in my life (in that order) I might find peace at last, and somebody to share my adventures with.

I still find I have sleepless nights; the jolly old brain tries to run when the body is walking, or maybe resting. I do hope I will find peace with someone at long last.

Chapter Twenty-One
TOTAL SHOCK

On Sunday, 5 May I thought I had completed my book in freehand. In fact, I thought I had completed it at 3 a.m. this morning. After receiving acupuncture treatment on Thursday, 2 May 2002, my ankle had a lot more mobility. This was the first day in thirty years that I did not have the feeling that I must go outside and be seen to be working to prove myself. I decided I would take it easy; I had been up till 3 a.m. this morning completing *Another World* and decided thirty years of a pathetic leg and arm being greatly improved deserved a rest.

I had been unable to wear sandals for the last thirty years due to the fact that my ankle was set in such a position that I continually tripped over the toe of my left sandal.

I had bought a new pair of sandals in Spain six weeks ago, they do not cost as much money in Spain, and every little thing helps. I thought, as my ankle has much more movement in it, that if I tried wearing the sandals at home on the flat surfaces of a carpet I would find it a lot of easier and hopefully not keep tripping over. I fitted them on. To my amazement and disbelief, I felt and observed four toes on my left foot move – this was the first time for thirty years and six weeks! I could not believe it. I knew I'd a few brandies last night. I said, 'Well, who woke you today, my little friends?' They did not utter a sound... What a surprise, tears started to flow. I went to my bedroom and curled up on my large twin bed, and I eventually started to cry.

I lay there for half an hour, shaking and crying with great relief. Fancy crying about my toes! It meant so much to me. My toes had been like a solid piece of rubber ever since the accident. Now with a lot of strengthening exercises and swimming I might at long last have a respectable body. It was too much for me, meeting Becky and my toes leaping back into your world. Would

I hopefully create a body not to be ashamed of and no longer feel inferior?

On Tuesday, 7 May 2002 I was selected to play for Rugby bowls team. Rugby Town's opponents were North Kilworth, who were a talented village team. It was unbelievable to walk into the club with two reasonably good ankles. I offered to buy a drink for all the players – I think that is going down in the Club's history book. My team-mates could not believe I was buying drinks, they thought there must be a catch; they were all fantastic about my achievements. I had an unbelievable game of bowls. It did not matter how I bowled the woods they seemed to go directly towards the white jack. I asked the Club Secretary, Spencer Pritchard, if they could find a vacant Friday evening so I could hold a BBQ, to thank all the bowlers for their great understanding over the last twenty years; also I could invite some close friends who had helped me. I would use it as a charity function to raise money for the Intensive Treatment Unit at Northampton and the Headway Charity.

Maybe the reason I get great enjoyment out of completing a challenge, and then moving on, is that I am showing people that persons with a disability or who are recovering from head-injuries are not as pathetic and incapable as they might appear. I wonder if other people feel inferior after suffering the same injuries as I did before 5 May 2002 when my toes came back into my life. I would love to know or maybe I ought to set up a confession group for people with such disabilities to explain how they feel about their condition.

I am sure a part of my recovery has been helped by my sometimes bluntly explaining in my book how I feel about various people and objectives. The movements of my toes instantly made the inferiority complex disappear. Also I have stopped lying. In the past when questioned how I was, rather than trying to explain how I felt about my disabilities which few people would understand, I just said, 'I am okay, thank you.'

Chiropractic treatment started in February 2001. Using the PAM started the thigh muscles working again on my left leg. Consistent physio most days in my life has eventually proved justified. I did these exercises at home, not as some people thought to save money, but because I felt too inferior to be amongst able-bodied people. Acupuncture has certainly been a revolution to my life; it has virtually stopped the severe pain in my right temple, which I had for thirty years. It has straightened my goofy left arm and helped my ankle regain flexibility and, of course, my toes to work. As I write this on 20 May 2002, tears are dropping on to the writing paper. What a softy – it is just so unbelievable!

After the initial shock of my little friends moving, I decided to start extra work in the gym. After two weeks I found this was too much for the brain to cope with as I began having mild headaches, of which previously I had few. Also, my body found the extra work too much; it was struggling to cope with the extra muscles working after such a long period dead.

It was October 2002 before I felt I was capable of returning to the work in the gym. I hope by May 2003 my physical state will be much improved. My mental state and speech have improved as I add these details on 13 November 2002.

A Young Lad

I want to tell you about a lad
Who had a problem
But his problem he would not discuss
He would lie awake most nights and wonder

He looked quite well
He wished he did not look that well
He had received quite a blow

Would he admit he was low? No
He was not beaten, but just going slow
His leg hurt every day
But give up he would not
Giving up was not in his vocabulary

His arm was bent, his leg very slow
This to people did not matter
But to him it was a flaw and quite a disgrace
And this made him feel quite incomplete

This lad was me. I cried with relief
And did not die
Motivating people is my life now
I think I will succeed – I know I will –
Thank you so much for my life
I hope I can help everybody a little.

Chapter Twenty-Two
MADEIRA

IN 1984 DILYS, THE LADY I WAS LIVING WITH, AND I DECIDED to take a holiday abroad. Due to the busy farming life that I was involved in with my brother and father, I did not get a lot of time off for holidays. We elected to spend a week in Madeira, the island of flowers and romance.

On holiday in Madeira I was chatted up by a timeshare lady; this was great. She was selling timeshares in one of the Pestana's hotels. Pestana's are one of the largest hotel resorts on the island. I decided that if I purchased two weeks in the timeshare apartment it would encourage me to come on a holiday more frequently. Unfortunately, as I became more involved with the farming I was unable to use my two weeks on the island.

Madeira is not large – thirty-six miles across – and it has wonderful *Levada* walks and unbelievable species of flowers. Funchal, the main town in Madeira, is the only flat spot in Madeira, down opposite the harbour. The warm climate and continuous walks up and down the slopes played a great part in my increasing strength in my left leg.

The Portuguese are wonderfully helpful and sociable people; nothing is too much for them to do to help you. The tourist industry has certainly put Madeira into the 2002 era. Certainly the town life has been modernised, but the rural hill life is still very much behind modern farming methods due to the lack of money and also the very mountainous landscape.

I have met some very loyal people in Madeira and made some good friends. As I write this chapter on Friday, 24 May, I am sitting in a covered area with large paned windows looking out at the beautiful clean blue sea. It is 72° outside; the sun is strongest between 12 a.m. and 3 p.m. I try and get out to the pool from 9 a.m. to 11 a.m; this time works in nicely with my typist, Irene, a tremendously attractive young Spanish lady. I believe she has an amazing multilingual capacity, five to six languages: tremendous! I can just cope with English and occasional Spanish or easy Portuguese words. We English are tremendously lazy. Most countries are English-speaking, as the English language is now international.

Irene has been the main person to type my book and this chapter. I never thought typing the book would be such fun; Irene finds my accent difficult to get a grip of (she can grip me any time – sorry, Irene). I must ask her if she minds me including that in my book. She has such a great sense of humour and we share a lot of laughs.

When I dictated my book, Irene often misunderstood: *brown* became *brnn*, *catch* became *cutch*, and so on, I have never laughed so much as when I have been attempting to write this book.

We think we might write a book about writing a book; it could be the greatest comedy ever dictated by an English/Spanish partnership. I think also by the time I finish the book in two weeks' time, Irene will be either insane or put off me completely because she will know my complete views on life and relationships (scary).

To be in the marketing business would be an ideal partnership with Irene (gosh, she has just thrown a fit, covered me with a glass of water and left for France – joke, I hope).

I find getting away to Spain or Madeira the ideal place to put my thoughts down in a reasonable order. There are no distractions apart from some gorgeous young Spanish, Portuguese, Brazilian and Italian ladies. I can cope with that, I have found, as this is my first book to be attempted. You just can't pre-book a time when you will feel like sitting down and putting your thoughts to paper.

Today, 24 May, as I write this chapter, it has been four days since I could sit down and put my thoughts of my past years to paper. Irene has just called me on my new mobile phone – yes, this time I have got it switched on. I only used to receive calls from certain people. I had not purchased a phone for Madeira use for eighteen years, but as I like people to keep in touch with me I had to buy a phone, because my UK phone would not function.

It has been quite a nice feeling, being out of contact with most people, but I do like people being able to contact me to offer me a meal. Irene phones to ask when I would be requiring her; I could have said tonight at 10 p.m., but I respect her and do not want a black eye. I respect and thank Irene so much for her tremendous skill at languages, her attempt at listening to someone with my strange feelings, such as I have expressed, and also for her valuable time. I think my business skills could be greatly improved with the help of my typist (that sounds selfish).

Now I will try to sell Madeira to you. Every island has its own cliché, and Madeira's is fortified wine production. The all-year-round mild climate has resulted in Madeira's elaborate nickname, 'The pearl of the Atlantic'. The first word that walkers might learn in Portuguese is *Levada*. *Levada* walking is unique to Madeira. Narrow irrigation channels cover the whole of the island in a cleverly devised network. These *Levadas* channel the water all over the island. The walks go by them.

With the latest laying of a lawn bowls green there will be something extra for the large majority of the holidaymakers. I have been wanting them to have one of these for the last five years. Oh well, in Portuguese style we have achieved it very quickly. Madeira Resorts Palace has these facilities and I would think that there will soon be more bowling greens. The present bowling green has only recently been laid. Unfortunately, only two rinks – Rome was not built in a day!

As I am a keen bowler, I will try and encourage bowlers to come from Warwickshire county. I play for Rugby Bowling Club in Warwickshire. I will encourage all my club members to visit Madeira to enjoy the tropical experience and also to enjoy an evening game of bowls. For the younger holidaymakers, there are wonderful waters where they can ski, scuba-dive, paraglide and sail. Nightlife is enjoyed in many Madeira bars. There are eight night-clubs in Funchal; they are all within walking distance of the centre. If you are staying in a hotel in the countryside there are plenty of taxis available which do not charge exorbitant prices.

Madeira

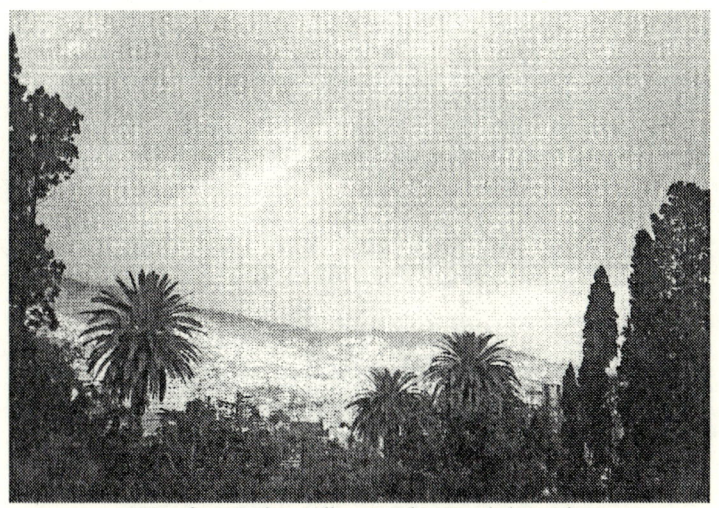

— View from Carlton Village Hotel in Funchal at night —

Complete

For thirty years
It was a struggle
I felt inferior and incomplete

It seemed every day
Was a complete struggle
Just to survive every stride
May 2002 – what a shock –
Acupuncture since February
Physio since August last
I had written a book
That was a surprise

My four toes could move
They wouldn't tell me why –
Do you know what I did?
Only cry
And say *Why*…

Complete at last
Inferior? Not now…
The world is my oyster
Motivate I will

For ever till I die
Thank you
For my sense of humour
Goodbye, inferior
Hello, complete.

12 June 2002

Thoughts

I thought we would play good bowls
I thought too much
Rocket as lead, it should be a good game
I at number two for a good result
Star at number three never there
At number four, the Skip he was a yard on

What a complete thought but what a day
Rocket could not see
When he did he was on the next rink
I followed Rocket to the bar.
Star, we thought, which year we still can not tell
The Skip, well he had a love affair with
The ditch, the woods or he were constantly
In the ditch

At the break it got better
All four were there
Liquid food and football to watch
The weather. It rained and rained, quite unfair

I pushed the curtain back to look outside
All I could see was, no window but a dartboard
The story of the day, it was never there.
It was nice to be there with my friends,
Ron, Ian K, and John C.
Thank you. Being there was a complete day
For me.
It is nice to be alive.

Chapter Twenty-Three
EMOTIONAL BREAK

IT IS QUITE WEIRD HOW THINGS WORK OUT. I HAD A BUSINESS meeting planned in Madeira for the last six weeks, and the length of this business meeting was, unusually, two weeks rather than one. This two-week break came at a very important point of my emotional recovery with my four toes leaping back to life. Yes, you may ask what is so emotional about the toes working again! Well, it was nearly too much for me. My words, however written, even by my gorgeous, considerate typist, cannot explain how I feel. I would not wish it on my worst enemy, to have suffered my last thirty years.

Thus the planned break in Madeira came fifteen days after the miracle (well, *I* think it was a bloody miracle).

For a change of airports I was leaving from Gatwick at 6 a.m. on 20 May. To save any delays on the early morning train I decided to take the 4 p.m. train the previous day.

So here was another of my little adventures; I had to make two changes to connect with my train to Gatwick. This went ahead quite nicely. When I arrived at Gatwick station, I followed signs for the taxi rank; this route took me into a lift: how nice, I have not got to carry my large suitcase up the sixty steps.

I manoeuvred my suitcase and briefcase into the lift, pressing hopefully the right button to take me upwards to the taxi rank. I should think I had been in the lift for forty seconds when suddenly we became stationary; I thought it would be just a split-second delay. Ten minutes later I was still stationary. At least the lift was, but I was not. I had tried pressing every button in the lift. I called emergency release but still remained stationary. I was just getting a little worried, when the next minute I saw a metal bar coming between the two lift doors. It seemed I had been jammed between two floors and the emergency team were having to open the lift doors manually.

I booked in at Moat House Lodge which was very comfortable. I had an early morning call at 3 a.m. and boarded my aircraft at 5.30 a.m. The flight was very comfortable; I was sat next to a couple with three children, aged between three and twelve, and their nanny. It proved to be a very entertaining flight.

When I arrived at the airport in Madeira, the person who had arranged to collect me was unavoidably detained, so I was lucky enough to get a nice female taxi driver to take me to my hotel. My hotel's name was the Imperatriz. This was a hotel I had stayed in before; it was situated between the old and new Funchal, ideal for business meetings all over the town. The staff were very helpful, even to the extent of making a pot of tea with a box of English tea I had taken with me. English tea in Funchal is like gold.

The second week I spent at the Oasis Atlantic, which is situated at the bottom end of Canico Baixo. This hotel is twenty-five minutes' drive from Funchal and has 224 rooms. The view from the turquoise-roofed hotel was unbelievable. It is only forty yards from the sea and at night you can hear the waves hitting the dark blue rocks and pebbles. It is so romantic – in my opinion the most romantic venue in Canico Baixo. The hotel provides many classes of restaurant meals. It has an outdoor swimming pool with heated sea water, another indoor pool and a children's swimming pool too. All rooms have partial or full sea view; there are daily entertainments and special nights at the Cocktail Bar.

My apartment had a direct view of the sea. When I opened my door into my bedroom I found it was massive in size; I would say it was thirty feet long by fifteen feet. As you entered the door on the left, there was a nice sized bathroom with a white bath and an overhead shower. It had a good-sized mirror and everything else you would expect. The apartment also contained a small kitchen, a cooker, a microwave and a fridge. There was a wonderful large built-in wardrobe, which would hold two people's clothes, plus your luggage. The ceiling and walls were white. The carpet was a slightly lighter blue than the sea colour with faint white diamond shapes. It was a wonderful bedroom, and all I needed was somebody to keep me company; but never mind, life goes on, thank goodness.

The two-week break was necessary for me firstly to finish off my work here and secondly to cope with the fantastic last four weeks. It has been a life challenge. Never ever did I think that my body would ever become respectable again – as I think it will in twelve months' time – and also not feel inferior to everyone else.

I will not stop now as I want to get my book printed and start on my motivation tour of the world. My main concern is to help, firstly, the victims of head-injuries and, secondly, and just as important, the parents who have to stand back and give respect to the victims and let them help themselves.

I have already arranged for barbecues and functions to raise money for a group called Headway, an organisation in Northampton for head-injury victims such as myself.

I must thank all my friends in Madeira for their loyalty and friendship. They accept me as a person with a limp and a goofy arm – they have never known me as anything else.

Lastly, and not least, I would like to thank Irene for her care and sensitivity dealing with my awful writing and the fact the computer we are writing on seems to have its own mind. It has taken us ten minutes to write the last two lines.

I do hope that this book helps somebody to laugh at their own situation and in turn aid their recovery. Also, I hope it will help you understand how some people feel after being struck such a vicious blow that nearly ended their life.

If only I can raise a smile or a chuckle from either a victim or parents who have been involved in similar incidents...

All I wish is to give people hope for the future.

Well, Becky is out of my life at the moment. Unfortunately Becky had to return to Ireland, in fact to Cork, with her mother to her mother's old home. Becky's father's death, as expected, has taken a lot out of the lives of Becky and family. Hopefully a visit and stay in the old home will help to heal the severe wound that has been left. I do not know when Becky will be back in England, or if she will stop in Ireland; either way I will be there for whatever she needs.

It is time to look for another challenge that will stop me becoming just a number that is counted but not appreciated.

Prepare myself for my last rugger game, motivation to go around the world and give hope to other victims when they have heard me describe my experiences and read *Another World*.

Well, I must now start to look for a gorgeous young lady to share my experiences and my adventures; she must also have a weird sense of humour because of my own very dry humour and thoughts.

To My Friends

Do not weep when I die
I will pay for a party when I die
To celebrate our lives shared.
Remember our struggle to survive
Our life's route not perfect, but with such love
I will protect you from above
In time you will join me
But I will never die
Nope, never die: I will be there to help you.

Chapter Twenty-Four
MY NEW LIFE

I AM A LITTLE UNSURE HOW TO DESCRIBE MY NEW LIFE. IT IS A similar life, but so different. It's 16 June 2002 and I am writing this while lying in bed – at four in the morning. That is why when dictating my early morning scribble it is taking quite a while.

All the thirty years since my ill-advised encounter with a motor vehicle and the initial darkness of life, I have being telling lies. When asked, 'How are you?' I have answered, 'Fine.' Inwardly I was so alone. Possibly because I had nobody from my world with whom I could discuss my feelings, as only they would understand my situation. Weird.

When I talk to people now I have nothing to hide. I played in a bowls gala. A gala, for those that are not involved in the world of bowls, is planned this way. You play eight ends, or for one hour, against a team of four players. The number of players can vary from gala to gala. After playing the first session you have one hour's rest. You then repeat this order four times. At the end of your four games the top four teams gaining the highest amount of points play for first, second, third or fourth position. The gala can take up to eight hours to complete.

My team of four players were playing together for the first time. Ron at lead; well, due to the rain, his glasses often were steamed up. This I decided was the reason he was seldom bowling his wood near to the jack. It rained all day. We were playing at Oakfield Bowling Club in Rugby. I played as number two position; I have played better. Ian K played as number three, we have named him 'Star'. The thing is we do not know when he was a star or will be a star. On the evidence of that day he might have to wait a long while. At number four position John played. He had, or his bowls had, a love affair with the ditch, because it seems his woods were always in the ditch.

My New Life

As the day got better, our game did not. We drew one and lost two by one shot or one bowl. The biggest defeat was by the runners-up of the gala. At our break for lunch, my team and I went to the clubhouse, which was only fifty yards from the bowling green. The lunch was mainly a liquid lunch, and so we could watch the World Cup on the TV, we sat down in the clubhouse by the outer wall. As it had been raining all day, I decided to pull back the curtain to see if it was still raining. Well, to my utter surprise, there was no window, but a dartboard. I asked, 'Who has stolen the window?'

It seems the curtain was there to cover the dartboard when not in use. I think the whole day the story had been, 'never there': firstly our woods were seldom near the white jack, and secondly the window was never there. What an extremely nice day.

What happened to me next I will never forget. A young lady by the name of Wendy had sponsored the gala. I had noticed this lady, as she was very attractive and made a nice change from looking at my bowling partners. She had shoulder-length auburn hair and a wonderful figure. She was presenting the first four awards to the winning teams.

Well, I thought, I have had an immensely good day and considered I deserved a prize, due to my recent astonishing event of my toes jumping back to life and having a most enjoyable day of bowls. I decided to ask her if being placed tenth in the gala deserved a kiss. Well, she was a complete lady with her attractive – I think greeny-brown – eyes, I cannot remember exactly the details as she gave me a wonderful long, time-consuming kiss.

That was the most cherished prize I have ever received for my bowls. Thank you, Wendy, I must thank Rocket Ron, the Star, Ian K, and the love-affair Skip, for a memorable day of bowls. How nice to be alive, able to walk and talk.

This afternoon I am playing for Rugby Town Bowling Club against Warwickshire Middleton bowling team. It will be an enjoyable day, rain or snow. I wonder if I can achieve tenth place and collect my award of a kiss? Certainly not from the President of our bowling club; he wears the wrong aftershave!

Chapter Twenty-Five
HEADWAY

HEADWAY IS A NATIONAL CHARITABLE ORGANISATION founded twenty years ago. It is for brain-injured people and their relatives. The work Headway achieves is unbelievable and often thankless.

I visited the club on 17 June 2002 at its new venue. It was the open day, and I wanted to surprise the organisers. The six clients – 'We call the patients clients out of respect to them.' – were tremendously interested to hear the details of my long recovery. I must say for one and a half hours I had their complete attention. It was nice for them to speak to somebody who had been in a similar condition to them. One of the clients said they had got more satisfaction from listening to me than from doctors in the last two years. It was a wonderful feeling for me that my thirty-year battle in 'Another World' was proving an incentive for other people.

This has certainly given my idea of going on a motivation talk a large incentive.

Billy, a client at Headway and a very attractive young lady, has a great interest in the world of sheep. We have a great deal of similar ideas. I suggested to them, when it eventually stops raining in Northamptonshire, that they all could come over to my farm for a picnic. This seemed to get a terrific response from the clients.

I suggest that for people to understand head-injured victims, they tie one hand behind their back and strap one leg to the other; this would give them a sure period of frustration when trying to complete a routine job. This will represent not just the frustration – sometimes lifelong – of head-injury victims but also other limb-restricting illnesses. Headway is in need of donations to help the running of the organisation, especially to follow down the road of acupuncture – which is, in my mind, the right direction for many people on the road to recovery.

It seems we can hand out money to people from other countries but cannot give money to our own countrymen who are living a very long, frustrating and sometimes empty life. Please, visit Headway, tie your hand or leg and try to complete your work...

See, how it frustrates you. Now who needs the money – maybe you? Think a little and then act. In one second you could be put into a head-injury trauma, and then what do you do. Your speech has gone, you cannot explain, your legs are useless and your side has gone. You realise now, but is it too late, it is never too late, I am the living proof.

I am donating 40% of the profit from *Another World* to the Headway charitable organisation for Northampton clients.

Further copies and information are available on:
www.athenapress.com

Friends

We are here to celebrate our lives
Remember, we all struggle at times
Love is needed to help our passage through life
So please do not query my funny shape
I am here to help you on your way
So please do not give up with a single sigh
Please give me a call and we will try again –
Thank you all for giving me your precious time.

Help

I am lost
I need some help
I was on my way to college
I received a blow

A head blow
Headway will help
Margo will be there
To help me through

I know what I want
But cannot tell
My voice has gone
But stress has not
Headway will help –
The charity for head-injuries

Who will help Headway?
Without some money Headway cannot survive
The work they do
Is so correct and unbelievable

Please judge not
Before you have had a look
Consider yourself in my state
Tie your hand behind your back
Strap one leg to the other
This might help you understand
How I feel
Money I need, *not* sympathy,
Fair play, help, understand
Please Help *Me*.

Postscript
THIRTY-TWO YEARS

In September 2004 I purchased a Niagara Hand Cycle Massage Unit – 75. I purchased this to massage my feet to improve circulation. I applied this to my feet – soles, heels and ankles – and my complete legs, from bottom to top. After three weeks my ankles had more movement and also my knees. It gave great relief to my right leg as this had, for many years, taken all the weight that my left leg was unable to support.

On 4th November 2004, when in Madeira on business organising the first ever Lawn Bowls Team to tour Madeira, I felt pins and needles in the sole of my left foot. I soon realised it was the nerves in my foot returning. (Speechless again!) Since that day my left leg has become more muscular.

Ian Litchfield, 2005

Printed in the United Kingdom
by Lightning Source UK Ltd.
116972UKS00001B/292-306